Periodontal Management of
Children, Adolescents and Young Adults

Quintessentials of Dental Practice – 17
Periodontology - 4

Periodontal Management of

Children, Adolescents and Young Adults

By
Valerie Clerehugh
Aradhna Tugnait
Iain L C Chapple

Editor-in-Chief: Nairn H F Wilson
Editor Periodontology: Iain L C Chapple

Quintessence Publishing Co. Ltd.

London, Berlin, Chicago, Copenhagen, Paris, Milan, Barcelona,
Istanbul, São Paulo, Tokyo, New Dehli, Moscow, Prague, Warsaw

British Library Cataloguing in Publication Data

Clerehugh, Valerie
    Periodontal management of children, adolescents and young adults. –
    (Quintessentials of dental practice. Periodontology ; 4)
    1. Pediatric periodontics
    I. Title II. Tugnait, Aradhna III. Chapple, Iain L. (Iain Leslie) IV. Wilson, Nairn H. F.
    617.6'32'0083

    ISBN 1850970718

Copyright © 2004 Quintessence Publishing Co. Ltd., London

Age icons and Fig 10-4 by Laura Andrew.

ISBN 1-85097-071-8

This book is dedicated to Tony and Mary with my love.
Val Clerehugh

Foreword

Many young people have periodontal problems which if overlooked or inappropriately managed may adversely influence the prognosis of the dentition. This latest addition to the *Quintessentials of Dental Practice* series provides a practical, well-illustrated guide to the aetiology, screening and diagnosis of periodontal diseases which may affect children, adolescents and young adults.

The values of teamwork, effective communication and knowing when to treat and when to refer to a specialist periodontist are rightfully stressed as important elements of the take-home message of this expertly crafted book. Owning and reading this *Quintessentials* book will be a pleasure, and then to go on to apply the enormous amount of evidence-based advice captured between the covers of this volume will, in all probability, transform the periodontal management of the children, adolescents and young adults you treat in your clinical practice.

As you would expect of a book in the *Quintessentials of Dental Practice* series, *Periodontal Management of Children, Adolescents and Young Adults* is an attractive publication written in a style aimed to appeal to busy practitioners and students. This book is an important volume in the series, and a valuable addition to dental literature in general. This is a book you will be very pleased to have read and to have available for ready reference.

Nairn Wilson
Editor-in-Chief

Preface

This is the fourth of five books in a series designed to provide the general dental practitioner with a contemporary, practical, illustrated guide for the management of patients with gingival and periodontal diseases. Our aim is to make the reader aware of the many and varied periodontal problems that can affect the young patient from childhood through to young adulthood and to provide a simple step-by-step approach to periodontal diagnosis and management in this group of patients. The need to look actively, and routinely, for periodontal disorders in these patients underpins our philosophy for their overall periodontal care. The role of the general dental practitioner in reaching an accurate diagnosis based on current disease classifications, in particular, is crucial to arranging appropriate treatment. Furthermore, the value of teamwork and good communication cannot be overemphasised, including an awareness of when to treat or when to refer to a specialist periodontist. The take-home message is that many young people really do have periodontal problems that can be easily missed unless appropriate screening is routinely undertaken to detect them and that the general dental practitioner has an important role in their management.

Having Read This Book

It is hoped that having read this book the reader will:

- Appreciate that a variety of periodontal problems can affect children, adolescents and young adults.
- Understand the key features of the periodontium in health and disease in the younger patient.
- Become familiar with the current classification of the periodontal diseases and be aware of how common or uncommon the various periodontal problems are in the younger patient.
- Appreciate that chronic periodontal destruction can begin in adolescence and that severe, aggressive forms of periodontal disease can affect children, adolescents and young adults.
- Understand the aetiology of the periodontal diseases and the interplay between the host defence systems and microbial plaque.
- Be aware of the nature of the local and systemic risk factors for periodontal diseases in the younger age groups.

- Be aware of the concept of periodontal risk at four levels: the patient, the mouth, the tooth and the specific site.
- Be knowledgeable about the rationale and methods of screening young patients quickly and simply for periodontal problems.
- Know how to reach a periodontal diagnosis in the younger age groups.
- Understand the principles of treatment planning and the three key stages of periodontal care.
- Appreciate the role of the dental team and the value of effective communication in periodontal patient management of children, adolescents and young adults.
- Appreciate the key stages in making a decision on whether to treat or refer a young patient for specialist periodontal care.

Valerie Clerehugh
Aradhna Tugnait
Iain LC Chapple

Acknowledgements

This book was written with the help and support of a number of people to whom we extend our grateful thanks: the Photography Department at Leeds Dental Institute for their photographic expertise; Multimedia Services at Birmingham's Dental School; Dr Simon Wood and colleagues in Oral Biology for kind permission to use Fig 2-3, and the *Journal of Dental Research* for permission to reprint it.

We would like to thank Stephen Fayle for Fig 5-5; Jack Toumba for Fig 10-5; Lesley Bensley for Fig 8-6; and Mike, Katy and Chloe Ehrlich for Fig 8-5; George Warman Publications (UK) Ltd for kindly granting us permission to reprint Figs 1-15, 5-5, 5-10 – 5-12, 6-10, 6-29, 7-7, 7-8, 9-1 – 9-3; Don Glenwright for Figs 6-1, 6-2, 6-4, 6-7, 6-25, 6-26; and Mosby Year Book for Figs 6-7, 6-11 and 6-13. We would also like to thank Maggie Jackson who devised the interdental brushes and kindly supplied Fig 8-9 and Professor Andy Blinkhorn for the oral health promotion leaflets that he so graciously provided for Chapter 9.

Dr Val Clerehugh wishes to say a huge thank you to her husband Tony and daughter Mary for their love, support and forbearance during the preparation of this book, and always. She also wishes to thank her mum, dad and her family for their unconditional support and guidance.

Dr Aradhna Tugnait wishes to thank her husband Keith for his loving support and his encouragement in the writing of this text and Mum, Anuja and Carl for always being there.

Professor Iain Chapple wishes to thank his wife Liz for her patience and unconditional support and little Jessica for giving up her valuable play time during the preparation of this fourth book.

Contents

Chapter 1
Periodontal Problems in the Young: Myth or Reality?

Aim

This chapter aims to dispel the myth that periodontal diseases are only of concern for adults in their thirties and older (Box 1-1). It provides an overview of the features of the different periodontal problems that can affect children, adolescents and young adults.

Outcome

After reading this chapter, the practitioner should be able to describe the features of periodontal health and diseases affecting the young patient during childhood, adolescence and young adulthood and be able to classify the different types of periodontal disease affecting this group of patients. They should also be aware of the epidemiology of key periodontal conditions affecting young patients.

Box 1-1

Myth or Reality?

Q. Is it myth or reality that periodontitis only affects adults after 30 years of age?

A. Myth!

Q. Is it myth or reality that periodontitis affects some children?

A. Reality!

Q. Is it myth or reality that periodontitis affects many teenagers?

A. Reality!

Q. Is it myth or reality that periodontitis affects young adults under 30 years of age?

A. Reality!

Q. Is it myth or reality that the current classification of periodontitis (International Workshop 1999) recognises a variety of periodontal problems that can affect young people under 30 years of age?

A. Reality!

READ ON . . .

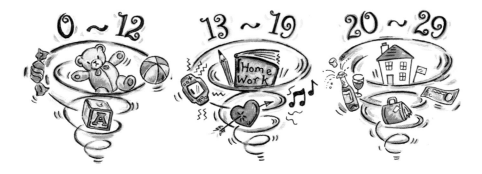

Fig 1-1 The three age groups of young patients: child, adolescent and young adult.

Children, Adolescents and Young Adults

As depicted in Fig 1-1, for the purposes of this text:
Children are: 0 – 12 years of age.
Adolescents are: 13 – 19 years of age.
Young adults are: 20 – 29 years of age.

Key Features of the Periodontium in Health

Appreciation of the key clinical and histopathological features of the periodontium in health is fundamental to the subsequent understanding of the disease process (Figs 1-2 and 1-3). For a more detailed account, the reader should refer to the first book in this series *Understanding Periodontal Diseases: Assessment and Diagnostic Procedures in Practice* (Chapple and Gilbert 2002).

The principal components of the periodontium are:
• gingiva (including epithelium and connective tissues)
• periodontal ligament
• cementum
• alveolar bone.

Gingiva

The healthy gingiva has a firm, pink, scalloped, knife-edged appearance, although pigmentation is a normal characteristic of certain ethnic groups. In the healthy state in children and teenagers, the gingival margin is several millimetres coronal to the cemento-enamel junction (CEJ). The gingival sulcus is essentially a shallow groove, 0.5–3mm deep on a fully erupted tooth,

2

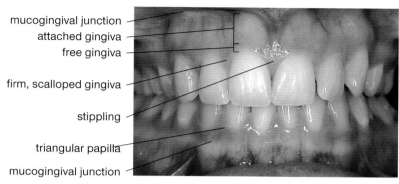

mucogingival junction
attached gingiva
free gingiva

firm, scalloped gingiva

stippling

triangular papilla

mucogingival junction

Fig 1-2 Healthy gingiva in a 21-year-old young adult.

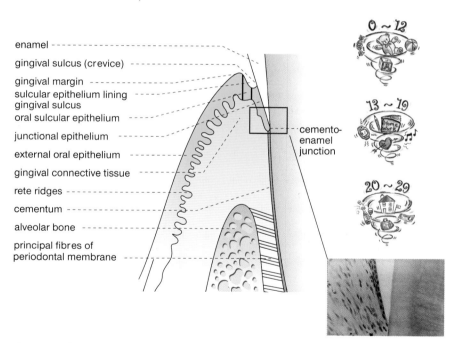

enamel

gingival sulcus (crevice)

gingival margin
sulcular epithelium lining
gingival sulcus
oral sulcular epithelium

junctional epithelium

external oral epithelium

gingival connective tissue

rete ridges

cementum

alveolar bone

principal fibres of
periodontal membrane

cemento-
enamel
junction

Fig 1-3 Schematic view of key features of periodontal health. Photomicrograph shows junctional epithelium. Note how widely spaced the cells are and how they thin out forming a single "terminal cell" layer at the apex of the junctional epithelium. Base of junctional epithelium is confluent with the most coronal connective tissue attachment level at the cemento-enamel junction.

3

which surrounds the tooth. It is lined by sulcular epithelium (SE) and junctional epithelium (JE), with the gingival margin forming its most coronal boundary (see Fig 1-3).

The gingiva attaches to the enamel via a weak junctional epithelial attachment, comprising the hemidesmosomes within the JE cells and a basal lamina that is produced by the epithelial cells. The hemidesmosomes attach the JE cells to the basal lamina, which in turn attaches to the tooth enamel. The cells of the JE attach to each other via desmosomes and gap junctions (Fig 1-4). JE is permeable with wide intercellular spaces, making it a leaky tissue through which various cells and substances transmigrate; for example, bacterial toxins may pass into the periodontal tissues and polymorphonuclear leucocytes (PMNLs) readily migrate from the tissues into the gingival sulcus as part of the first line of the periodontal host defence system (see Chapter 2). The JE is also weak and is readily disrupted by periodontal probing or flossing which can cause it to split. The split occurs within the JE, rather than between the JE and enamel; fortunately, this is soon repaired (two to six days) due to the rapid turnover of epithelial cells. The most coronal surface of the JE forms the base of the gingival sulcus, where it is approximately 0.15mm wide and comprises 20 – 30 cell layers. The most apical extent of normal, healthy JE is usually at the CEJ and is only a single cell layer wide (see Figs 1-3 and 1-4).

The presence of a plaque-free zone (PFZ) corresponding to the JE was first

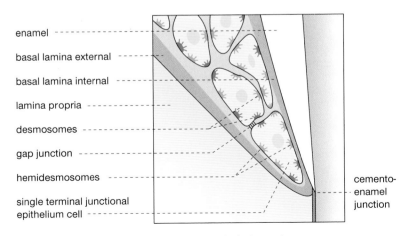

Fig 1-4 Schematic diagram of junctional epithelial attachment.

reported to be present on extracted teeth in the 1940s. Subsequent studies demonstrated that three zones can be identified within this PFZ: a narrow, permeable coronal zone with few JE cell remnants, a middle adhesive zone where many JE cell remnants are visible and an apical zone in which the JE cells have germinative characteristics. The studies showed that the width of the JE is variable, and that it is widest around the molars and narrowest around incisors. The JE generally decreases as the loss of attachment (LOA) and pocket depth increase. The base of the JE is confluent with the most coronal extent of the periodontal connective tissue attachment level, an important landmark (Fig 1-3).

In children free from periodontal disease, it would be expected that the periodontal connective tissue attachment level would be at the CEJ on the fully erupted tooth and that the epithelial attachment would be located on enamel. The molar tooth in Fig 1-5, extracted due to caries in a teenager, has been stained with Gomori's stain for one minute. Two grooves can be seen that mark the gingival margin mid-buccally and mesiobuccally prior to extraction. Supragingival plaque is evident on the crown of the tooth that has a wide PFZ corresponding to the previous location of the JE. A band of adhesive JE cell remnants in the middle of the PFZ is visible. After extraction, some of the periodontal fibres remain in the tooth socket while the rest adhere to the tooth root. It can be seen that the periodontal fibres are attached right up to the CEJ, showing that there has been no LOA. This healthy status can be maintained through the teenage years to adulthood (see Fig 1-3).

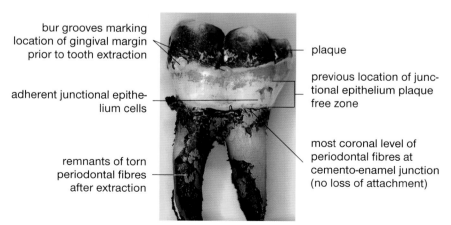

bur grooves marking location of gingival margin prior to tooth extraction

plaque

previous location of junctional epithelium plaque free zone

adherent junctional epithelium cells

remnants of torn periodontal fibres after extraction

most coronal level of periodontal fibres at cemento-enamel junction (no loss of attachment)

Fig 1-5 Plaque-free zone on extracted molar tooth stained with Gomori's stain.

5

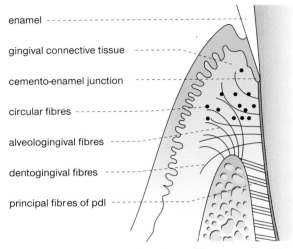

enamel

gingival connective tissue

cemento-enamel junction

circular fibres

alveologingival fibres

dentogingival fibres

principal fibres of pdl

Fig 1-6 Schematic view of principal collagen fibre groups of the connective tissues of the gingiva.

Connective Tissue

The predominant tissues of the gingiva and periodontal ligament are the connective tissues that principally comprise collagen fibres (60%), with fibroblasts (5%), blood and lymph vessels, nerves and extracellular matrix forming the rest. The gingival collagen fibres are organised into bundles, which are named according to their course and insertion (Figs 1-6 and 1-7):

- dentogingival fibres
- alveologingival (alveolar crest) fibres
- circular fibres
- transseptal fibres.

Periodontal Ligament

The periodontal ligament (PDL) has several functions, the most important being to provide attachment between the root cementum and alveolar bone. It resists the forces applied to the tooth and thus protects the nerves and blood vessels at the root apex from damage during function. The PDL is responsible for the mechanisms by which the tooth attains and maintains its functional position after eruption, including the phenomenon of tooth drifting that may occur as a consequence of periodontal destruction. Cells from the PDL have a role in the formation, maintenance and remodelling of alveolar bone and cementum. Mechanoreceptors in the PDL provide sensory input for reflex jaw activities.

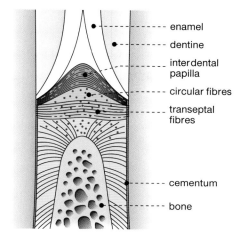

enamel

dentine

interdental papilla

circular fibres

transeptal fibres

cementum

bone

Fig 1-7 Schematic view of the interdental area showing the transseptal fibres and a cross-section of the circular fibres.

The periodontal ligament fibres (Fig 1-8) are grouped into:
• alveolar crest fibres
• horizontal fibres
• oblique fibres
• apical fibres.

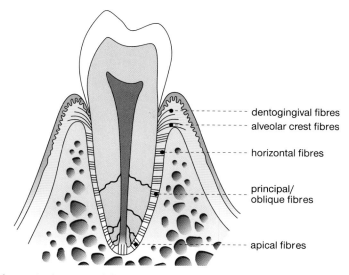

dentogingival fibres

alveolar crest fibres

horizontal fibres

principal/ oblique fibres

apical fibres

Fig 1-8 Schematic diagram of the periodontal ligament.

7

The portions of the principal periodontal ligament fibres that are embedded in the cementum and alveolar bone are called Sharpey's fibres.

Cementum

Cementum can be classified into two types according to the presence or absence of cells (Fig 1-9):

1. Acellular (primary) cementum forms on the root dentine during root formation and tooth eruption. Mineralised Sharpey's fibres form a large proportion of acellular cementum.
2. Cellular (secondary) cementum contains cementocytes in lacunae and canaliculi and forms after tooth eruption in response to function. It usually overlies the acellular cementum in the apical area of the root where the cementum layer is generally thicker (0.2–1.0mm) than in the coronal part of the root (0.05–0.10mm).

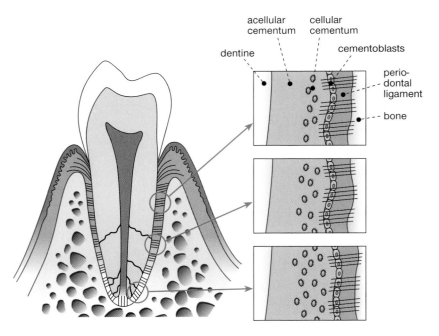

Fig 1-9 Schematic view of basic cementum structure. Note that the cementum layer becomes thicker and more cellular towards the tooth apex.

Alveolar Bone

The alveolar bone is that part of the maxilla or mandible that supports and protects the teeth. There are two types of bone: compact (cortical) bone is dense and solid; spongy (cancellous) bone contains a lattice of bony trabeculae. The external and internal alveolar plates on both the buccal and the lingual surfaces are formed of compact bone, while in between is a variable amount of spongy bone. Posteriorly, the external alveolar plate is 1.5–3.0mm thick but is thinner and more variable around the anterior teeth. The thickest cortical bone is on the buccal aspect of the mandibular molars, whereas the thinnest is on the mandibular incisors. This anatomical variation accounts for two clinical phenomena.

1. It influences the ability of local anaesthetic solution to permeate the alveolus to reach the nerves supplying the anterior and posterior teeth in the mandible and maxilla. It is also one of the factors that influences the choice of local anaesthetic technique for periodontal therapy (see Chapter 8 and also Meechan 2002).
2. The thinness of bone in the lower incisor region predisposes to the development of bony fenestrations (windows in the bone), and dehiscences (gaps in the bone) which, in turn, may be associated with recession of the overlying gingiva (Fig 1-10).

The tooth sockets are lined by a thin layer of compact bone that provides attachment to some of the principal periodontal ligament fibres. Radiographically, this bone appears as a dense white line that is called "lamina dura". Studies carried out by Clerehugh's group (in conjunction with Haus-

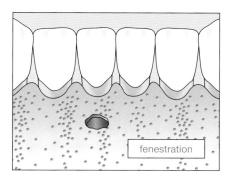
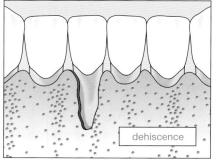

Fig 1-10 Schematic diagram of bony fenestration and dehiscence.

mann's team in Buffalo, USA) have shown that in healthy teenage subjects with no clinical loss of attachment, the alveolar crest is situated between 0.4mm and 1.9mm apical to the CEJ.

Key Features of Gingivitis

Plaque-induced gingivitis is characterised by micro-ulceration of the JE, inflammatory cell infiltration of the connective tissue, lateral proliferation of the JE and formation of rete ridges. It can occur at any age from childhood, through teenage years and young adulthood, to beyond (Fig 1-11). As the supragingival plaque accumulates, so the inflammatory infiltrate increases and attachment between the enamel and the JE weakens. This allows migration of the plaque in an apical direction with deepening of the gingival sulcus and extension of the plaque subgingivally. In this way a gingival pocket forms. The most apical extent of the JE is still, however, at the CEJ, no LOA has occurred and the alveolar bone is still intact. This process is entirely reversible provided the aetiological agent, plaque, is removed.

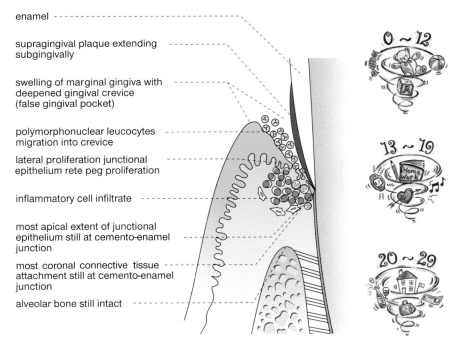

enamel

supragingival plaque extending subgingivally

swelling of marginal gingiva with deepened gingival crevice (false gingival pocket)

polymorphonuclear leucocytes migration into crevice

lateral proliferation junctional epithelium rete peg proliferation

inflammatory cell infiltrate

most apical extent of junctional epithelium still at cemento-enamel junction

most coronal connective tissue attachment still at cemento-enamel junction

alveolar bone still intact

Fig 1-11 Schematic view of the key features of gingivitis.

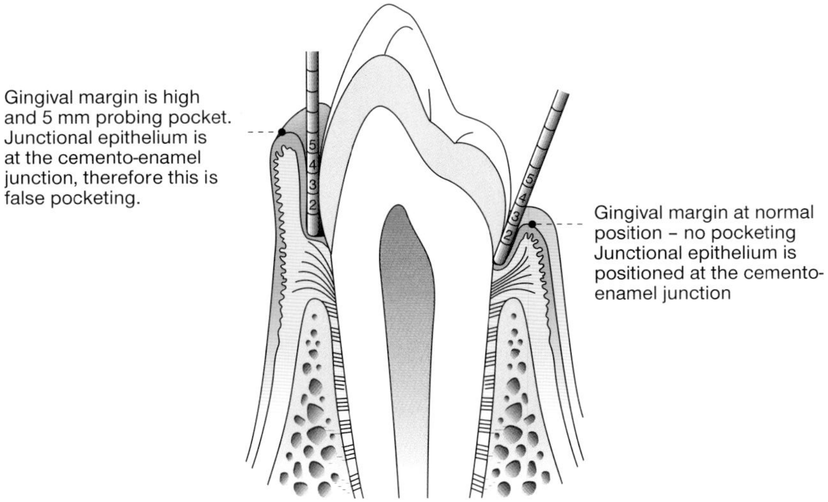

Gingival margin is high and 5 mm probing pocket. Junctional epithelium is at the cemento-enamel junction, therefore this is false pocketing.

Gingival margin at normal position – no pocketing Junctional epithelium is positioned at the cemento-enamel junction

Fig 1-12 Schematic longitudinal section of a premolar and associated periodontal tissues, demonstrating a healthy sulcus and false pocketing due to overgrowth of the gingiva.

A severe inflammatory process may be accompanied by swelling of the gingival margin, thereby creating a false gingival pocket over 3mm deep, i.e. the base of the pocket is still at the CEJ (Fig 1-12), and there has been no LOA or bone loss. Although gingivitis may remain stable for weeks, months, years or may never progress, some patients or sites may be at risk of progression to irreversible periodontitis for a variety of reasons (see Chapter 2).

Key Features of Periodontitis

There are three key features of periodontitis, irrespective of the type:
• Loss of attachment of the periodontal connective tissues to the cementum.
• Apical migration of the JE beyond the CEJ (clinical attachment level now apical to CEJ) and transformation of the JE to pocket epithelium which is often thin and ulcerated.
• Alveolar bone loss.

The transition from gingivitis to the initial stages of periodontitis (incipient

11

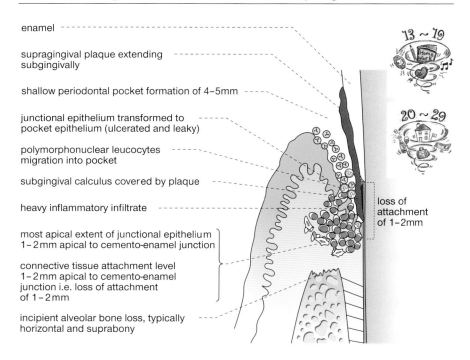

enamel

supragingival plaque extending subgingivally

shallow periodontal pocket formation of 4–5mm

junctional epithelium transformed to pocket epithelium (ulcerated and leaky)

polymorphonuclear leucocytes migration into pocket

subgingival calculus covered by plaque

heavy inflammatory infiltrate

most apical extent of junctional epithelium 1–2mm apical to cemento-enamel junction

connective tissue attachment level 1–2mm apical to cemento-enamel junction i.e. loss of attachment of 1–2mm

incipient alveolar bone loss, typically horizontal and suprabony

loss of attachment of 1–2mm

Fig 1-13 Schematic view of key features of incipient periodontitis that can occur at interproximal sites during the teenage years and later.

chronic periodontitis) is not just confined to adults but can and does happen in many teenagers. Initial periodontal destruction is characterised by 1–2mm interproximal LOA, formation of true periodontal pockets 4–5mm deep and crestal alveolar bone loss of about 0.5mm, which is typically horizontal (Fig 1-13). This form of periodontitis usually progresses relatively slowly throughout the teenage years into young adulthood and beyond, although local and systemic factors can influence the rate, severity and extent of progression.

Although relatively uncommon, some very advanced, aggressive forms of periodontitis can affect children, teenagers and young adults. These severe forms of destruction are characterised by interproximal LOA of at least 3mm, (often much more), deep periodontal pockets of 6mm or greater, plus alveolar bone loss which is typically vertical/infrabony, (Fig 1-14) although the precise presentation depends on the aetiology and type of periodontitis.

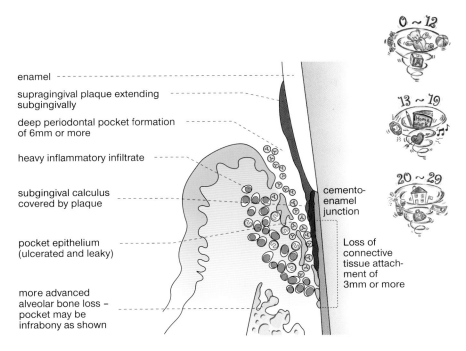

enamel

supragingival plaque extending
subgingivally

deep periodontal pocket formation
of 6mm or more

heavy inflammatory infiltrate

subgingival calculus
covered by plaque

pocket epithelium
(ulcerated and leaky)

more advanced
alveolar bone loss –
pocket may be
infrabony as shown

cemento-
enamel
junction

Loss of
connective
tissue attach-
ment of
3mm or more

Fig 1-14 Schematic view of key features of advanced periodontitis. These features are typical of aggressive forms of periodontitis that can affect a small proportion of teenagers or young adults. Although uncommon, certain systemic diseases can also give rise to such advanced lesions in children.

Classification of Periodontal Diseases in Children, Teenagers and Young Adults

Classification of Gingivitis

An International Workshop for the Classification of Periodontal Diseases and Conditions took place in 1999. The full classification is shown in Table 1-1. For a detailed account of the background to the debate, the rationale behind the final consensus and a critique of this latest classification, the reader is referred to Chapple and Gilbert (2002). The next section highlights the key aspects of the classification as applied to children, teenagers and young adults. Application of the classification during clinical diagnosis, with a précis of the clinical and radiographic features, is covered in Chapter 5.

Table 1–1 Classification of periodontal diseases proposed by the International Workshop (1999)

A. Dental plaque-induced gingival diseases

1. Gingivitis associated with dental plaque only
   a. without other local contributing factors
   b. with local contributing factors

2. Gingival diseases modified by systemic factors
   a. associated with the endocrine system
      1) puberty-associated gingivitis
      2) menstrual cycle-associated gingivitis
      3) pregnancy-associated
         a) gingivitis
         b) pyogenic granuloma
      4) diabetes mellitus-associated gingivitis
   b. associated with blood dyscrasias
      1) leukaemia-associated gingivitis
      2) other

3. Gingival diseases modified by medications
   a. drug-influenced gingival diseases
      1) drug-influenced gingival enlargements
      2) drug-influenced gingivitis
         a) oral contraceptive-associated gingivitis
         b) other

4. Gingival diseases modified by malnutrition
   a. ascorbic acid-deficiency gingivitis
   b. other

B. Non-plaque-induced gingival lesions

1. Gingival diseases of specific bacterial origin
   a. *Neisseria gonorrhea*-associated lesions
   b. *Treponema pallidum*-associated lesions
   c. streptococcal sp.-associated lesions
   d. other

2. Gingival diseases of viral origin
   a. herpes virus infections
      1) primary herpetic gingivostomatitis
      2) recurrent oral herpes
      3) varicella zoster infections
   b. other

3. Gingival diseases of fungal origin
   a. *Candida* sp. infections
      1) generalised gingival candidosis
      2) linear gingival erythema
      3) histoplasmosis
      4) other

4. Gingival lesions of genetic origin
   a. hereditary gingival fibromatosis
   b. other

5. Gingival manifestations of systemic conditions
   a. mucocutaneous disorders
      1) lichen planus
      2) pemphigoid
      3) pemphigus vulgaris
      4) erythema multiforme
      5) lupus erythematosus
      6) drug-induced
      7) other
   b. allergic reactions
      1) dental restorative materials
         i)   mercury
         ii) nickel
         iii) acrylic
         iv) other
      2) reactions attributable to
         i)   toothpastes/dentifrices
         ii) mouthrinses/mouthwashes
         iii) chewing gum additives
         iv) foods and additives
      3) other

6. Traumatic lesions (factitious, iatrogenic, accidental)
   a. chemical injury
   b. physical injury
   c. thermal injury

7. Foreign body reactions

8. Not otherwise specified (NOS)

contd.

C. Chronic periodontitis
1. Localised
2. Generalised

D. Aggressive periodontitis
1. Localised
2. Generalised

E. Periodontitis as a manifestation of systemic diseases
1. Associated with haematological disorders
  a. acquired neutropenia
  b. leukaemias
  c. other

2. Associated with genetic disorders
  a. familial and cyclic neutropenia
  b. Down syndrome
  c. leucocyte adhesion deficiency syndromes
  d. Papillon-Lefèvre syndrome
  e. Chédiak-Higashi syndrome
  f. histiocytosis syndromes
  g. glycogen storage disease
  h. infantile genetic agranulocytosis
  i. Cohen syndrome
  j. Ehlers–Danlos syndrome (types IV and VIII)
  k. hypophosphatasia
  l. other

3. Not otherwise specified (NOS)

F. Necrotising periodontal diseases
1. Necrotising ulcerative gingivitis (NUG)
2. Necrotising ulcerative periodontitis (NUP)

G. Abscesses of the periodontium
1. Gingival abscess
2. Periodontal abscess
3. Pericoronal abscess

H. Periodontitis associated with endodontic lesions
1. Combined periodontic-endodontic lesions

I. Developmental or acquired deformities and conditions

1. Localised tooth-related factors that modify or predispose to plaque-induced gingival diseases/periodontitis
   a. tooth anatomic factors
   b. dental restorations/appliances
   c. root fractures
   d. cervical root resorption and cemental tears

2. Mucogingival deformities and conditions around teeth
   a. gingival/soft tissue recession
      1) facial or lingual surfaces
      2) interproximal (papillary)
   b. lack of keratinised gingiva
   c. decreased vestibular depth
   d. aberrant fraenum/muscle position
   e. gingival excess
      1) pseudopocket
      2) inconsistent gingival margin
      3) excessive gingival display
      4) gingival enlargement
   f. abnormal colour

3. Mucogingival deformities and conditions on edentulous ridges
   a. vertical and/or horizontal ridge deficiency
   b. lack of gingiva/keratinised tissue
   c. gingival/soft tissue enlargement
   d. aberrant fraenum/muscle position
   e. decreased vestibular depth
   f. abnormal colour

4. Occlusal trauma
   a. primary occlusal trauma
   b. secondary occlusal trauma

Source: Adapted from Chapple and Gilbert, Understanding Periodontal Diseases: Assessment and Diagnostic Procedures in Practice. London: Quintessence, 2002; 1999 International Workshop for a Classification of Periodontal Diseases and Conditions. Ann Periodontol 1999;4:1–112.

Gingivitis was included in the 1999 classification, in contrast to previous classifications. The plaque-induced gingival diseases are very common in all age groups, and Table 1-1 shows the many forms of the disease that can present in daily dental practice. It is important to be aware that modifying factors can come into play that have the potential to influence the natural course and management of a particular gingival disease. It is also worth bearing in mind that while the classic description of plaque-induced gingivitis is as depicted in Chapter 5 (Box 5-1), where there has been no LOA, it can also occur on a periodontium with reduced support in which the attachment loss and bone loss has stabilised and is not progressing. Modifying factors that influence the natural course of the disease and risk factors that increase the susceptibility of the child to gingival problems can be identified from the history and examination of the young person as outlined in Chapters 2 – 4. Less commonly, non-plaque-induced gingival lesions can present in the young. Since the diagnosis and management of some of these are challenging, Chapter 6 is devoted to this topic.

Classification of Periodontitis
Chronic periodontitis
It is significant that the terminology has changed from "adult periodontitis" to "chronic periodontitis" (Table 1-1) as this heralds the increased international awareness that periodontitis is not just confined to adults in their thirties, and beyond, but can begin in adolescents and progress throughout the teens, as shown by Clerehugh and co-workers in the 1990s (Clerehugh, *et al*. 1990, 1995, 1997). Progression into young adulthood and beyond is common. The destruction resulting from chronic periodontitis is consistent with the microbial aetiology of the disease in the presence of local risk factors (such as plaque-retentive restoration overhangs) and/or systemic factors (such as smoking, stress or poorly controlled diabetes mellitus).

Aggressive periodontitis
The replacement of the previous term "early onset periodontitis" by "aggressive periodontitis" helps to impress a rapidly destructive disease without undue emphasis being placed on the age of presentation, albeit a disease that usually, but not exclusively, affects young adults under the age of 30 years. It is a distinct and separate entity from chronic periodontitis and must be managed differently.

Common features of aggressive periodontitis are:
• Patient clinically healthy (apart from the presence of periodontitis).

- Rapid LOA and bone destruction.
- Familial aggregation.

Secondary features (not always present) are:
- Amount of microbial deposits inconsistent with severity of periodontal destruction.
- ↑ numbers of *Actinobacillus actinomycetemcomitans*
  – in some populations may be ↑ *Porphyromonas gingivalis*.
- Phagocyte abnormalities (especially PMNL, see Chapter 2).
- Hyperresponsive macrophage phenotype, including ↑ prostaglandin E_2, interleukin-1β.
- Progression of LOA and bone loss may be self-limiting.

Periodontitis as a manifestation of systemic diseases
Poorly controlled diabetes and tobacco smoking have not been included in this section of the 1999 classification since both can be significant modifiers of all forms of periodontitis. Rather, the expert panel that drew up this section included systemic diseases of which periodontitis is a frequent manifestation. Many of these are rare (e.g. Papillon-Lefèvre syndrome, Chédiak-Higashi syndrome) and will be briefly discussed in Chapter 7.

Most of the young patients with severe periodontal destruction of their deciduous dentitions who were previously classified as having "pre-pubertal periodontitis" would now be included in this section. Therefore, the term pre-pubertal periodontitis was excluded from the 1999 classification. Any young child with periodontal destruction in the absence of systemic factors should be classified under chronic periodontitis or aggressive periodontitis, as appropriate. Evidence from retrospective epidemiological data has shown radiographic bone loss around the primary dentition in some children, reinforcing the notion that periodontitis can develop at an early age and further dispelling the myth that it is a disease only affecting adults.

Periodontitis associated with endodontic lesions
This category recognises the interaction of the periodontal and endodontic pathologies, irrespective of the primary source of infection, as demonstrated by Chapple and Lumley in early 1999 (see Chapter 5).

Necrotising periodontal diseases
Necrotising periodontal diseases were grouped together in the 1999 classification to encompass the conditions necrotising ulcerative gingivitis (NUG) and necrotising ulcerative periodontitis (NUP), the latter probably a con-

tinuum of the former. NUG is uncommon among Western European populations (0.001% of British and Danish populations), but is more common in developing countries such as Nigeria, NUP is rare but it is believed to occur more frequently in HIV-positive individuals. Progression of NUP to cancrum oris has been reported in malnourished children and to necrotising stomatitis in immunosuppressed individuals.

Classification of abscesses
In the 1999 classification, abscesses were classified as either gingival, periodontal, pericoronal or associated with endodontic lesions. The descriptor "lateral" was omitted from the previous nomenclature lateral periodontal abscess, so that this is now simply a periodontal abscess.

Epidemiology of Chronic Periodontitis and Aggressive Periodontitis

The study of periodontal epidemiology in the younger age groups has been hampered by lack of agreed periodontal criteria, but recent major reviews have addressed many of these issues and concluded that significant localised or generalised periodontal problems can affect the mixed and permanent dentitions (Jenkins and Papapanou 2001, Albandar and Tinoco 2002).

Incipient Chronic Periodontitis
The initial, "incipient" stage of periodontal destruction in a young patient will typically be characterised by loss of periodontal connective tissue attachment (LOA) of 1–2mm, formation of true shallow periodontal pockets of 4–5mm, and early crestal alveolar bone loss of at least 0.5mm. Clerehugh and co-workers have performed validity studies to demonstrate that with a careful technique it is feasible to detect low thresholds of disease, namely LOA of up to 3mm. This involves the so-called "one-stage" LOA measuring technique whereby the probe tip is located at the CEJ using tactile sensation, and the tip advanced apically until the clinical attachment level is reached (i.e. base of pocket), whilst at the same time directly observing the distance, in millimetres, advanced by the probe (Fig 1-15).

A five-year longitudinal study of 167 teenagers in North-West England by Clerehugh *et al.* (1990) showed the prevalence of LOA of 1mm increased from 3% at age 14 years to 37% at age 16 years and to 77% by age 19 years. At the 2mm threshold for LOA, none of the 14-year-olds were affected, but 3% of the 16-year-olds and 14% of the 19-year-olds had at least one site affected; however, only 3% of sites (examined using a partial recording sys-

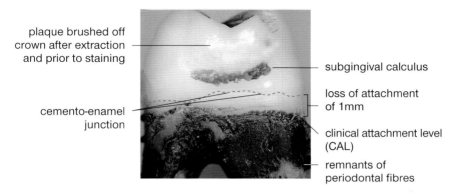

plaque brushed off
crown after extraction
and prior to staining

subgingival calculus

loss of attachment
of 1mm

cemento-enamel
junction

clinical attachment level
(CAL)

remnants of
periodontal fibres

Fig 1-15 Loss of periodontal connective tissue attachment (loss of attachment = 1mm) on a stained extracted maxillary molar tooth from an adolescent. Note: the plaque was brushed off, prior to staining, to facilitate observation of the clinical attachment level. See the calculus on the enamel that had been subgingival prior to extraction.

tem) had 2mm LOA in the 19-year-olds. The lower prevalence at this slightly more severe 2mm level is consistent with other epidemiological studies. Other key findings (Clerehugh, *et al.* 1990, 1995, 1997) are:

- Development of LOA was associated with the presence of subgingival calculus and supragingival plaque.
- Significantly more Indian and Pakistani teenagers were affected by chronic periodontitis than Caucasian teenagers.
- The subgingival plaque in affected subjects harboured a complex subgingival microflora including putative periodontal pathogens such as *P. gingivalis*, *P. intermedia* and *A. actinomycetemcomitans*.
- Prevalence of periodontitis varies according to the threshold set for disease and the ethnicity of the study group.

Aggressive Periodontitis

This form of periodontitis is much less common than chronic periodontitis, but the effects can be devastating due to the rapidity and severity of the periodontal destruction. The epidemiology of localised aggressive periodontitis (formerly localised juvenile periodontitis or localised early-onset periodontitis) has been well documented. It is estimated to affect 0.1–0.2% of Caucasians, in contrast to 2.6% of Blacks; there is no gender predisposition. It is more difficult to estimate the prevalence of the generalised form, but it is likely to affect less than 5% of the population. Both localised and generalised aggressive periodontitis (formerly generalised juvenile periodontitis or generalised early-onset periodontitis or rapidly progressive periodontitis) are likely to be encountered by the dental practitioner at some time.

Key Points

- Recognition of the features of the periodontium in health and disease in children, adolescents and young adults is important to understand the disease process.
- It is a myth that periodontitis does not affect children and adolescents.
- The 1999 periodontal disease classification outlines current consensus views of a large panel of international experts on classification of periodontal diseases and conditions.
- Many forms of periodontal diseases and conditions affect children, adolescents and young adults.
- Most are primarily plaque induced, but some forms of disease are not.
- In reality, chronic periodontitis begins in adolescents and is common. The prevalence, extent and severity slowly increase during teenage years.
- In reality, aggressive periodontitis is an uncommon but rapidly destructive disease that can severely affect adolescents and young adults, leading to tooth loss. Localised and generalised forms may occur.

References

Albandar JM, Tinoco EMB. Global epidemiology of periodontal diseases in young persons. Periodontol 2000. 2002;29:153–176.

Armitage GC. Development of a classification system for periodontal diseases and conditions. Ann Periodontol 1999;4:1–6.

Chapple ILC, Lumley PJ. The periodontal-endodontic interface. Dent Update 1999;26:331–341.

Chapple ILC. A whistle-stop tour of the periodontium. In: Chapple ILC, Gilbert AD. Understanding Periodontal Diseases: Assessment and Diagnostic Procedures in Practice. London: Quintessence, 2002:1–16.

Clerehugh V, Lennon MA, Worthington HV. 5-year results of a longitudinal study of early periodontitis in 14- to 19-year-old adolescents. J Clin Periodontol 1990;17:702–708.

Clerehugh V, Worthington HV, Lennon MA, Chandler R. Site progression of loss of attachment over 5 years in 14- to 19-year-old adolescents. J Clin Periodontol 1995;22:15–21.

Clerehugh V, Seymour GJ, Bird PS, Cullinan M, Drucker DB, Worthington HV. The detection of *Actinobacillus actinomycetemcomitans, Porphyromonas gingivalis* and *Prevotella intermedia* using an ELISA in an adolescent population with early periodontitis. J Clin Periodontol 1997;24:57–64.

Jenkins WMM, Papapanou PN. Epidemiology of periodontal disease in children and adolescents. Periodontol 2001;26:16–32.

Further Reading

1999 International Workshop for a Classification of Periodontal Diseases and Conditions. Ann Periodontol 1999;4:1–112.

Berkowitz BKB, Holland GR, Moxham BJ. Oral Anatomy, Histology and Embryology, 3rd edn. Edinburgh: Mosby, 2002.

Meechan JG. Practical Dental Local Anaesthesia. London: Quintessence, 2002.

Chapter 2

Development of Periodontal Diseases in the Younger Population

Aim

The aim of this chapter is to outline the defects in biological processes that may lead to the development of periodontal diseases in the younger population.

Outcome

After reading this chapter the practitioner should be able to appreciate that the balance between host defence mechanisms and microbial plaque influences periodontal disease outcome. The nature of plaque and what constitutes the host defence against microbial plaque should be clear. Susceptibility to disease is dependent on the interplay between a number of risk factors. The practitioner should be aware of these at all levels: the patient, the mouth, the individual tooth and the specific site. Finally, the transition from established gingivitis to periodontitis in the young patient should be understood.

Balance: Microbial Challenge Versus Host Defence

Whilst the microbial aetiology of gingivitis is not in any doubt, the transition from reversible plaque-induced gingivitis to irreversible periodontitis is unpredictable (Fig 2-1). In a balanced situation, the host's defence mechanisms can contain the pathogenic effects of the microbial plaque so that disease does not progress. If there are host defence problems, or there is a change in the quantity or quality of the microbial challenge, causing either end of the see-saw to tip, then the balance is upset and disease can progress resulting in periodontal tissue destruction (Fig 2-2).

The Nature of Plaque
Biofilm
Plaque is a biofilm comprising a complex microbial community in a matrix of polymers of bacterial and salivary origin. It has a complex three-dimensional structure that serves to protect it from the host's defence mechanisms and from antimicrobial agents (Fig 2-3). Supragingival plaque comprises approximately 50% matrix, and the plaque bacteria tend to be Gram-posi-

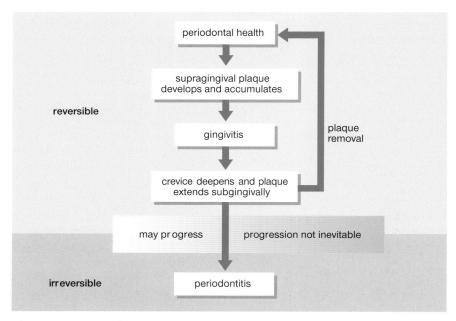

Fig 2-1 Transition from reversible gingivitis to irreversible periodontitis.

tive cocci and rods, which are largely aerobic unless the plaque layer is thick. In contrast, although it develops by extension from supragingival plaque, subgingival plaque has very little matrix, and survives at a much lower oxygen concentration. As the subgingival plaque matures in a highly anaerobic environment, the constituent microflora shifts and harbours an increasing proportion of Gram–negative rods and spirochaetes.

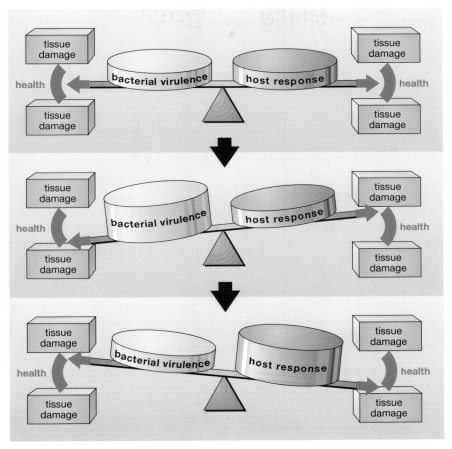

Fig 2-2 The delicate balance between microbial activity and host defences, which maintains periodontal tissue health. Such equilibrium may easily be disrupted, leading to inflammation and tissue damage.

Over 400 microbial species have been detected in the oral environment, but only a relatively small number have been specifically implicated in the periodontal disease process. There are three hypotheses of how plaque causes periodontal disease:

- Specific plaque hypothesis.
- Non-specific plaque hypothesis.
- Ecological plaque hypothesis.

27

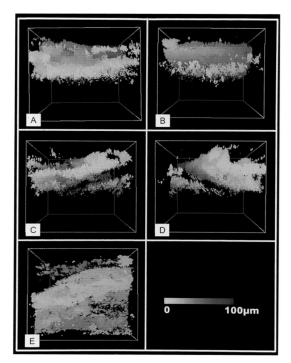

Fig 2-3 Biofilm: three-dimensional colour-coded reconstruction of intact human plaque based on a series of 200 xy reflectance images taken at 0.6μm intervals from the surface of the plaque to the enamel surface. Variations in plaque density are apparent and channels can be seen running through the biofilm (bright yellow, closest and dark red (100μm), distant).

Specific plaque hypothesis

According to this hypothesis, individual bacterial species are responsible for inflammatory periodontal disease, for example, as is the case with tuberculosis. Over a century ago, Koch put forward the postulates that set out the various requirements for microbial specificity to be attributed in a disease. Thus, in the specific plaque hypothesis, the clinical implications for periodontal treatment are two-fold:

• Treatment should be directed towards elimination of the pathogen and prevention of re-establishment.
• Plaque control would not be necessary, since plaque without the pathogen would be non-pathogenic.

Although several pathogens have been implicated since the 1990s (Box 2-1), none has satisfied all of Koch's postulates.

28

Box 2-1

Suspected Periodontal Pathogens

Actinobacillus actinomycetemcomitans

Bacteroides forsythus

Campylobacter rectus

Eikonella corrodens

Fusobacterium nucleatum

Porphyromonas gingivalis

Prevotella intermedia

Peptostreptococcus micros

Spirochaetes, *e.g. Treponema denticola*

Very few periodontal conditions are associated with specific pathogens. Nevertheless, *A. actinomycetemcomitans* has been strongly implicated in localised aggressive periodontitis. It possesses many virulence factors some of which are specifically designed to evade host defence systems. Elimination of *A. actinomycetemcomitans* can be difficult and often requires mechanical therapy with adjunctive systemic antibiotic treatment. Studies have shown that successful therapy is associated with elimination of this organism. Fusiforms, spirochaetes and *P. intermedia* have been associated with necrotising ulcerative gingivitis (NUG).

Non-specific plaque hypothesis
This hypothesis suggests that in the absence of effective plaque control, the indigenous plaque bacteria colonise the gingival sulcus and form plaque. Inflammatory periodontal disease develops when the combined effects of the total microbial challenge overcome the host's defence mechanisms. All plaque bacteria are thought to have some virulence factors capable of causing gingival inflammation and subsequently periodontal destruction. Implications for treatment are:
- Total plaque control is necessary in the prevention of the plaque-induced periodontal diseases.
- Patient's oral hygiene must be effective.
- Professional scaling and root surface debridement must be meticulous.

This hypothesis does not explain the variations in pathogenic potential or the different types of periodontal disease. It does not address why some patients never progress from gingivitis to periodontitis and why some sites remain stable while others progress. Its application, therefore, is limited to chronic gingivitis.

Ecological plaque hypothesis
Haffajee and colleagues in 1991, discussed an "environmental" plaque model and Marsh (1994) subsequently proposed that dental plaque forms naturally on the teeth and helps the host's defence systems by preventing colonisation of exogenous and often pathogenic (non-resident) species. Plaque accumulation around the gingival margin leads to an inflammatory response and increased gingival crevicular fluid flow, the constituents of which can affect the local environment and change the subgingival plaque ecology, this shifts from mainly Gram-positive to obligatory anaerobic asaccharolytic Gram-negative bacteria. When the microbial homeostasis is altered, these sites are susceptible to periodontal disease. The prevailing treatment consideration involves inhibition of periodontal pathogens:
• directly (by subduing the pathogens) or
• indirectly (by interfering with factors that drive the transition, e.g. use of anti-inflammatory drugs).

No single plaque hypothesis has so far been able to explain fully plaque's role in the disease process, but the ecological hypothesis is the one which most agree best fits chronic periodontitis.

Host defence systems

The young patient's defence mechanisms are critical, as they keep plaque bacteria and their products out of the periodontium and destroy any that do manage to get through. There are five key defence systems (Fig 2-4):
• saliva
• epithelium
• inflammatory response (innate immunity)
• immune response (acquired specific immunity)
• soluble mediators of the inflammatory immune response.

Saliva
Saliva protects only those parts of the periodontium where it can gain access within the so-called salivary domain. In contrast, host defence mechanisms in the gingival crevice and periodontal pocket are deemed to be in the crevic-

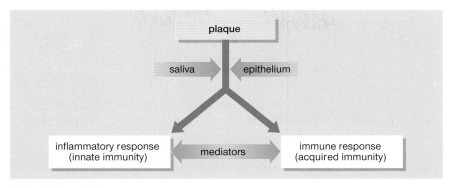

Fig 2-4 Host defences.

ular domain, as they are derived from the gingival crevicular fluid and inflammatory cells. Any defects or disturbances in these defence mechanisms will tip the balance (see Fig 2-2) and lead to periodontal destruction. Saliva has a number of important functions:

- washing effect
- vehicle for swallowing bacteria (10^8/ml of saliva)
- inhibition of bacterial attachment by secretory immunoglobulin (IgA)
- killing of bacteria by salivary peroxidase system
- other antimicrobial actions by various salivary components, e.g. lysozyme, lactoferrin.

Although saliva does not directly affect subgingival plaque constituents, lack of saliva (xerostomia) can be associated with supragingival plaque build up and the development of gingivitis. For example, youngsters who have lack of lip seal (incompetent lips) and breathe through their mouth may present with an exacerbation of their plaque-induced gingivitis anteriorly where the gingival tissues have dried out (Fig 2-5). Certain drugs may also adversely influence salivary flow, as can irradiation surgery involving the salivary glands. A variety of gingival problems and cervical caries may be an unfortunate consequence in some of these patients.

Epithelium
Intact epithelium is a physical barrier to the plaque micro-organisms. Once the junctional epithelium (JE) has transformed into pocket-lining epithelium, with its micro-ulcerations and leaky structure, its protective function is compromised. Epithelium can induce an inflammatory response via keratinocytes.

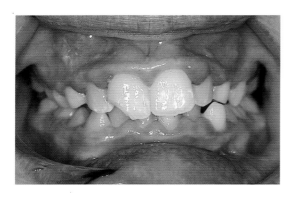

Fig 2-5 Plaque-induced gingivitis exacerbated anteriorly by lack of saliva in a 12-year-old boy who breathes through his mouth, with lack of lip seal (incompetent lips).

Langerhan's cells (tissue macrophages) trap antigens and present them to lymphocytes, thereby initiating the immune response (Fig 2-6).

Inflammatory response (innate immunity)
The inflammatory response is a non-specific response to microbial plaque antigens, which dilute or "wall off" the damaging agents and kill them. The response has two components:
• fluid response (tissue fluid and gingival crevicular fluid (GCF))
• cellular response polymorphonuclear leucocytes (PMNLs), macrophages, lymphocytes, platelets and fibroblasts).

The GCF washes non-adherent bacteria out of the crevice and contains mediators of inflammation, breakdown products (which are nutrients for plaque bacteria) and antibacterial agents (antibody, complement); flow increases with increasing inflammation.

The PMNLs are crucial cells in the inflammatory process and form the first line of defence. PMNLs are attracted down a chemical gradient towards the invading micro-organism (chemotaxis) (Fig 2-7). They recognise, bind to and kill bacteria with or without phagocytosis (whereby the bacteria are first engulfed and then destroyed). Specific adhesion molecules may assist the PMNLs' movement into the crevice by acting as cellular traffic controllers, e.g. ICAM1 (see Chapple and Gilbert 2002).

Macrophages have important functions in both the inflammatory process and the immune response. In inflammation, they phagocytose and kill bacteria. They modulate the fluid and cellular phases of inflammation and secrete mediators of inflammation. In addition, they remove damaged host tissue and secrete tissue-degrading enzymes.

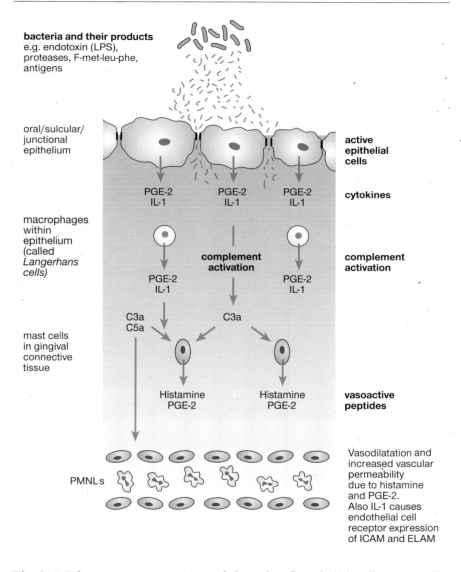

Fig 2-6 Schematic representation of the role of epithelial cells, mast cells, macrophages and complement in the production of cytokines and vasoactive peptides that produce key vascular changes in early inflammation.

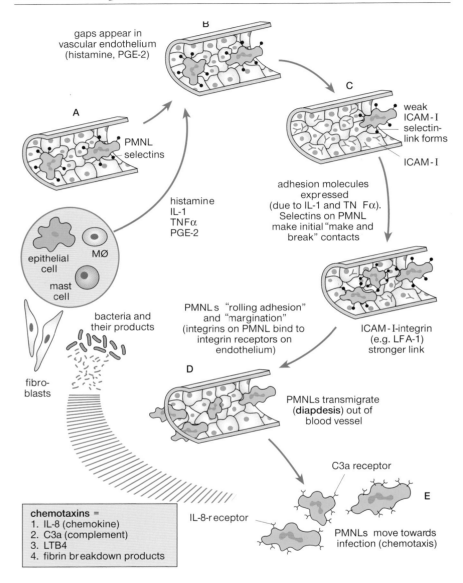

Fig 2-7 Schematic representation of the processes involved in the recruitment of neutrophils from blood vessels to sites of tissue damage and infection.

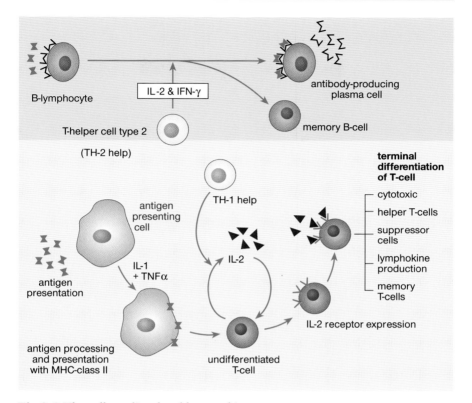

Fig 2-8 The cell-mediated and humoral immune responses.

Unfortunately, the powerful effects of the inflammatory process on the plaque antigens can induce by-stander damage on the neighbouring "innocent" tissues.

Immune response (acquired/specific immunity)
This is a highly specific response to the antigen and has the advantage that it has memory. There are two types of immune response (Fig 2-8):
• humoral
• cell–mediated.

The antigen (micro–organism) is recognised by lymphocytes that circulate continuously through the blood, lymphatics and tissues. Lymphocyte clonal expansion produces a larger pool of cells that differentiate to induce a humoral or cell–mediated response.

The **humoral** response is the most important response in the periodontal diseases (see Fig 2-8). Langerhan's cells in the epithelium take up the antigen, which is then carried to the lymph nodes and presented to the circulating lymphocytes. Following clonal expansion, the B-lymphocytes differentiate into plasma cells that secrete antibody (Immunoglobulin, "Ig") against the specific antigen (antibody generating) under the control of the T-lymphocytes (T-helper cells). Most of the antibody produced is IgG, while IgM plays a lesser role and is produced earlier in the infective process. The antibody may be produced systemically or locally and acts by:
- aggregating and clumping of molecules
- preventing microbes adhering to the epithelium
- working with complement to lyse microbes
- working with PMNLs to produce efficient opsonisation, phagocytosis and killing.

Although the precise mechanisms are unknown, the humoral response appears to be protective. In localised aggressive periodontitis, antibodies to *A.a.* are found, whereas in chronic periodontitis, antibodies to *P. gingivalis* are seen.

The **cell-mediated** response does not need an antibody (see Fig 2-8); the T-cell has its own receptor called the T-cell receptor. After stimulation by presentation of antigen, T-helper lymphocytes:
- produce cytokines
- assist the differentiation of B-lymphocytes into plasma cells
- activate PMNLs and macrophages.

Macrophages trap and present antigens to T-lymphocytes to induce an immune response in the connective tissues (not the gingival crevice), whilst adhesion molecules, e.g. CD44 act as "anchors". They also secrete interleukin-1 (IL-1) and tumour necrosis factor alpha (TNF-α) to promote an efficient response.

On the whole the cell-mediated response appears to contribute less to the host defence mechanisms than the humoral response. T-killer lymphocytes appear to play no role in periodontal defence.

Mediators
Mediators are soluble, chemical messengers that regulate/provide a link between the inflammatory response, the immune response and tissue damage. Their actions are short-lived, potent and subject to rapid inactivation.

They include:
- cytokines
  - interleukins (pro-inflammatory; transmit information between leucocytes)
  - TNF-α (pro-inflammatory)
  - transforming growth factor beta (TGF-β; both pro- and anti-inflammatory)
  - chemokines, e.g. IL-8
- prostaglandins, e.g. PGE_2 (bone resorption, neutrophil chemotaxis, vascular permeability and dilation)
- matrix metalloproteinases (MMPs; degrade connective tissue)
- complement (pro-inflammatory)
- histamine (vascular permeability and dilation).

Host Defence Defects in the Young Patient

Where there is a defect in the host defence system, the young patient is susceptible to more severe and rapid periodontal destruction than normal. Defects in PMNLs have been implicated in localised aggressive periodontitis and Down syndrome. Reductions in PMNL numbers in cyclic neutropenia and agranulocytosis predispose the patient to periodontal problems (see Chapters 6 and 7).

The generalised prepubertal periodontal breakdown found in children with leucocyte adhesion deficiency syndrome is linked to structural defects in their leucocytes that affect leucocyte adherence and subsequent migration into the blood stream. Chédiak-Higashi syndrome is another example of a neutrophil disorder predisposing the child to severe periodontal breakdown. Epithelial and connective tissue defects contribute to the devastating periodontal tissue destruction found in Papillon-Lefèvre syndrome. These will be covered more fully in Chapter 7.

Neutrophil and other host defence defects are also thought to play a role in the periodontal problems found in those with poorly controlled diabetes or in those who smoke cigarettes.

Genetic disorders

The host defence defects described above are believed to be genetic in origin. For example, the neutrophil defects of cyclic and chronic neutropenia are inherited as an autosomal dominant trait. In contrast, inheritance by autosomal recessive trait accounts for the neutrophil defects found in leucocyte adhesion deficiency syndrome, Chédiak-Higashi syndrome, glycogen storage disease 1b, infantile genetic agranulocytosis and Cohen's syndrome.

The epithelial/connective tissue defects found in Papillon-Lefèvre syndrome are acquired by autosomal recessive inheritance, whereas in Ehlers-Danlos syndrome, the defects are acquired by autosomal dominant inheritance.

A familial tendency has been reported in cases of aggressive periodontitis, although there is no consensus on the precise nature of inheritance.

Periodontal Disease Risk

Periodontal risk factors
Periodontal risk factors increase the likelihood of periodontal disease developing without necessarily being causal. There are two main categories:
- Systemic risk factors (see Chapter 3), including:
  - systemic diseases/conditions that affect host defence mechanisms (e.g. smoking, diabetes, stress)
  - host defence defects (e.g. Down syndrome).
- Local risk factors (see Chapter 4) that:
  - increase plaque retention, therefore increase microbial challenge, e.g. subgingival calculus
  - directly damage periodontal tissues (e.g. finger nail picking habit on gingival margin); Class II division 2 malocclusion in which the upper incisor(s) impinge on the lower labial gingiva.

Determining periodontal risk
The transition from health to disease or from a stable gingivitis to periodontitis occurs when the balance between the microbial challenge and host defence mechanisms is upset, i.e. when either the microbial challenge outweighs and overcomes the host defence mechanisms or when there are defects in the host response that allow the microbial challenge to effect damage (see Fig 2-2). Determination of periodontal risk in the younger patient can be undertaken at four levels (Fig 2-9):
- Patient level (e.g. systemic risk factors, genetic susceptibility, smoking).
- Mouth level (e.g. severity, extent and rapidity of periodontal destruction relative to age, oral hygiene, occlusion).
- Individual tooth level (e.g. bone support, mobility, drifting).
- Specific site level (e.g. attachment loss, pocket depth and presence of bleeding on probing at specific site, local root groove/concavity, suppuration).
Application of the risk assessment model is depicted in Fig 2-10.

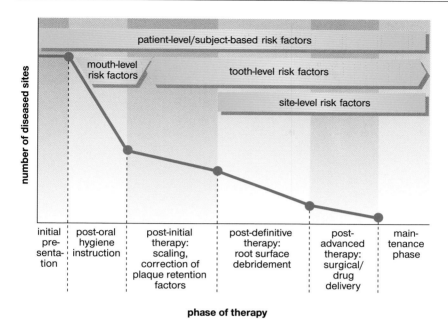

Fig 2-9 The potential effectiveness of different stages of periodontal therapy, and how levels of multiple risk assessment can apply to each stage.

PATIENT NAME:

REGISTRATION NO:

DATE OF BIRTH:

DIAGNOSIS: *Chronic incipient periodontitis*
(UR6, UL6, LL21 and LR12)

SYSTEMIC RISK FACTORS:

+ve family history ❑   Diabetes ❑
Smoker (pack years)_____   Stress ❑
Other _____

Fig 2-10 A simple tick-box system, which can be incorporated into an ink stamp to be placed in a susceptible patient's notes to record risk factors.

Development of Periodontitis in the Younger Age Groups

Initial Inflammation

The first signs of inflammation are seen 24–48 hours after supragingival plaque accumulation. The microbial products initiate a host response either through damage to the epithelium or because they are recognised by Langerhan's cells in the epithelium. The tissue damage leads to release of mediators of inflammation and an acute inflammatory response, in which vasodilation occurs and PMNLs are found in the gingival connective tissues subjacent to the junctional epithelium. PMNLs migrate to the gingival crevice. Antigenic bacterial factors initiate an immune response, which in turn triggers a more specific inflammatory response.

As an increasing number of plaque accumulates and extends subgingivally, the lesion develops and more inflammatory cells (including lymphocytes and macrophages) are recruited to the area. The immune response results in production of antibodies by plasma cells, and cytokines are released by epithelial cells, T-cells and macrophages. An increase in GCF flow occurs and there is continued migration of PMNLs into the gingival crevice. Swelling of the gingival tissues leads to deepening of the gingival crevice, which favours an anaerobic Gram-negative bacterial flora; more damaging factors are produced, e.g. endotoxin, proteolytic enzymes. Rete peg proliferation ensues in the most coronal junctional epithelium. Early loss of collagen is seen in the gingival connective tissue.

Established Gingivitis

The established gingivitis lesion (Fig 2-11) comprises a plasma cell dominated chronic inflammatory infiltrate. There is heavy PMNL migration into the gingival crevice. Extensive supragingival and subgingival plaque deposits can be found. Micro-ulceration of the JE makes this an ineffective barrier, but the passage of microbial products through it is hindered by the flushing action of the GCF; any that slip through are neutralised by the host defence mechanisms.

Importantly, there is no loss of periodontal connective tissue attachment and no alveolar bone loss. The equilibrium between the microbial plaque challenge and the host defence systems may continue. The established gingivitis lesion may resolve on removal of the plaque aetiological agent. Alternatively, there may be exacerbations, for example during a period of stress when host defence mechanisms and oral hygiene are both adversely compromised, leading to irreversible periodontal tissue breakdown.

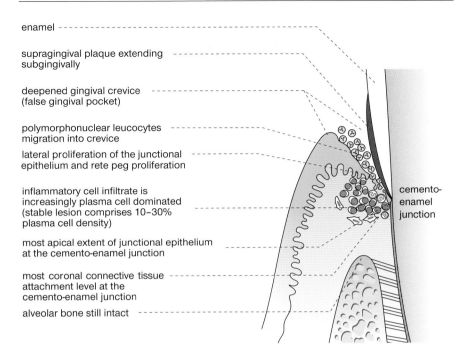

enamel

supragingival plaque extending subgingivally

deepened gingival crevice (false gingival pocket)

polymorphonuclear leucocytes migration into crevice

lateral proliferation of the junctional epithelium and rete peg proliferation

inflammatory cell infiltrate is increasingly plasma cell dominated (stable lesion comprises 10–30% plasma cell density)

most apical extent of junctional epithelium at the cemento-enamel junction

most coronal connective tissue attachment level at the cemento-enamel junction

alveolar bone still intact

cemento-enamel junction

Fig 2-11 Established gingivitis – the cellular and tissue level.

Periodontitis

There are similarities between the inflammatory infiltrate in the established gingivitis lesion and the chronic periodontitis lesion. It was hypothesised that development of periodontitis from gingivitis in children is accompanied by a change from a T-cell to a B-cell dominated lesion, though not all researchers agree. Currently there is consensus that plasma cells are the dominant cell type in periodontitis (Fig 2-12).

Frank periodontal breakdown occurs affecting the periodontal connective tissue attachment level and periodontal ligament. In the incipient chronic periodontitis lesion, often seen in adolescents, this connective tissue attachment level may be 1–2mm apical to the CEJ. Apical migration of the JE, now called pocket epithelium, leads to true periodontal pocket formation; such pockets are shallow (4–5mm) initially. Alveolar bone resorption occurs leading to bone loss.

41

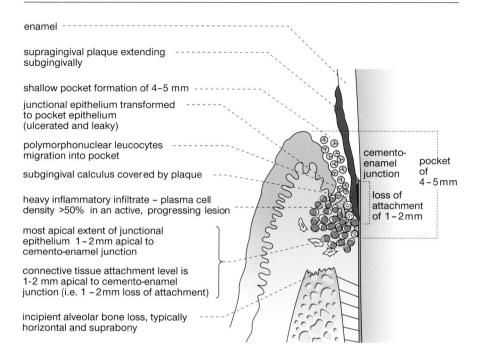

enamel

supragingival plaque extending
subgingivally

shallow pocket formation of 4–5 mm

junctional epithelium transformed
to pocket epithelium
(ulcerated and leaky)

polymorphonuclear leucocytes
migration into pocket

subgingival calculus covered by plaque

heavy inflammatory infiltrate – plasma cell
density >50% in an active, progressing lesion

most apical extent of junctional
epithelium 1–2 mm apical to
cemento-enamel junction

connective tissue attachment level is
1-2 mm apical to cemento-enamel
junction (i.e. 1 –2 mm loss of attachment)

incipient alveolar bone loss, typically
horizontal and suprabony

cemento-
enamel
junction

pocket
of
4–5 mm

loss of
attachment
of 1–2 mm

Fig 2-12 Incipient periodontitis – the cellular and tissue level.

Progression of the lesion may well lead to advanced periodontal destruction even in a teenager, in whom severe loss of attachment (LOA; in excess of 3mm) and deep pocketing (6mm or more) are typical features of aggressive periodontitis (Fig 2-13).

Key Points

- The balance between the microbial challenge and host defence mechanisms determines whether periodontal diseases develop, remain stable or progress.
- Plaque is a biofilm within which pathogens are protected.
- Plaque hypotheses (specific, non-specific, ecological) provide clues as to appropriate periodontal management.
- Host defence systems include saliva, epithelium, inflammatory response, immune response and soluble mediators of inflammatory-immune response.

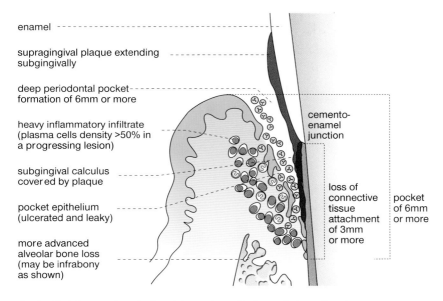

enamel

supragingival plaque extending subgingivally

deep periodontal pocket formation of 6mm or more

heavy inflammatory infiltrate (plasma cells density >50% in a progressing lesion)

subgingival calculus covered by plaque

pocket epithelium (ulcerated and leaky)

more advanced alveolar bone loss (may be infrabony as shown)

cemento-enamel junction

loss of connective tissue attachment of 3mm or more

pocket of 6mm or more

Fig 2-13 Advanced periodontitis – the cellular and tissue level.

- Systemic and local periodontal risk factors influence susceptibility to disease.
- Periodontal risk can be determined at four levels:
  - patient
  - mouth
  - individual tooth
  - specific site.
- Development of periodontitis can occur in the younger age groups but is not an inevitable progression from gingivitis.

References

Haffajee AD, Socransky SS, Smith C, Dibart S. Microbial risk indicators for periodontal attachment loss. J Periodont Res 1991;26:293–296.

Marsh PD. Microbial ecology of dental plaque and its significance in health and disease. Adv Dent Res 1994;8:263–271.

Further Reading

Chapple ILC. The role of the host response. In: Chapple ILC, Gilbert AD. Understanding Periodontal Diseases: Assessment and Diagnostic Procedures in Practice. London: Quintessence, 2002:31–49.

Hodge P, Michalowicz B. Genetic predisposition to periodontitis in children and young adults. Periodontol 2000. 2001;26:113–134.

Kinane DF, Podmore M, Ebersole J. Etiopathogenesis of periodontitis in children and adolescents. Periodontol 2000. 2001;26:54–91.

Williams DM, Hughes FJ, Odell EW, Farthing PM (Eds.) Pathology of Periodontal Disease. Oxford: Oxford University Press, 1992:67–97.

Chapter 3

History and Systemic Risk Factors for Periodontal Diseases

Aims

The aims of this chapter are two-fold: first, to outline the key aspects of history taking in child, adolescent and young adult patients with periodontal problems; and secondly, to identify the principal systemic periodontal risk factors in these age groups that may be identified from the history.

Outcomes

After reading this chapter the practitioner should be aware of the aspects of history taking that are relevant for periodontal diseases in the younger age groups and consent issues that may arise when dealing with young patients. The dentist should also be able to elicit systemic risk factors for periodontal diseases and appreciate the relevance of such information for the diagnosis of periodontal conditions in children, adolescents and young adults.

Consent

Adults

Adults are presumed competent to give their consent for examination or treatment unless demonstrated otherwise. If there are any doubts about this, the question to ask is "Can this patient understand and weigh up the information needed to make this decision?". This is an important issue because obtaining **informed consent** is based upon the patient making a decision to undertake treatment after having been provided with, and having understood, all benefits and risks of that treatment, and any alternatives.

Children

Before starting a consultation involving children, the clinician needs to be sure that the appropriate consent to examine or treat the child has been obtained. Most children will attend the dentist accompanied by an adult, but this may not always be the parent or guardian. It is important to determine the relationship between the child and accompanying adult so that an informed and reliable medical history can be taken and consent to treat can be given. At 16 years of age the patient is considered able to give their own consent although it may still be appropriate for parents or guardian to be involved and this may well be the adolescent's preference. Even though in the UK a child's consent can be valid if they are considered to be mature enough to understand the planned treatment, in most circumstances it is still prudent to include the parents or guardian in the discussion.

The History

The history enables the clinician to collect relevant personal details by interview, which will form the basis for the periodontal examination and in turn, the diagnosis of the periodontal condition. It is at this stage that the dentist will also begin to establish a professional relationship with the young adult, the teenager or the child and his or her parent, and will develop an impression of their health attitudes and any particular anxieties.

The history can be broadly divided into the following key areas (Fig 3-1), although the exact order of questioning is at the discretion of the individual dentist:

- Presenting complaint and history of complaint/reason for attendance.
- Family periodontal history.
- Medical history.
- Dental history.
- Social history.

Presenting Complaint and History of Complaint/Reason for Attendance

The reason for the patient's visit and any particular complaint, together with the history of the complaint should be elicited. If the patient has presented in pain then details of the nature of the pain, location, onset and duration should be recorded. In many cases the patient will present for a check-up without pain. Patients do not always report signs or symptoms of dental disease unless prompted so specific questions should be asked of the patient and parent or guardian: for instance whether their gums bleed on brushing or if any teeth are sensitive.

Family History of Periodontal Diseases

Some periodontal diseases have a familial association and the dental history of other members of the family may then be relevant and provide an indication about the likely natural history of the disease process. It is worth asking: "Is there a history of gum disease, pyorrhoea or early tooth loss in the family – brothers, sisters, parents or grandparents?".

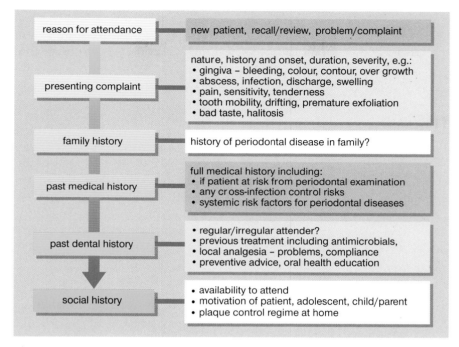

Fig 3-1 Key stages in the periodontal history taking of young patients.

Medical History

The medical history is important in identifying children, adolescents and young adults with medical problems who:

1. May be at risk when undergoing periodontal examination or treatment, due to:
   - a cardiac lesion
   - congenital heart disease
   - a confirmed significant heart murmur.

   These medical conditions may put the patient at risk of infective endocarditis from a bacteraemia resulting from invasive periodontal procedures (such as periodontal probing, scaling and polishing, subgingival instrumentation, root planing or extractions), unless prophylactic antibiotics are given in accordance with current recommended guidelines.

2. May pose a cross-infection control risk to dental professionals and subsequent patients, e.g. carriers of hepatitis B – such patients should be managed according to current local infection control guidelines.

47

3. May have a systemic factor that can increase the risk of the young patient having or developing periodontal disease. The following list is based on the categories proposed by Chapple and Gilbert (2002) but is limited to those conditions pertinent to children, adolescents and young adults:

A. Genetic/inherited/inborn risk factors (see Chapters 2, 6 and 7 for more detailed accounts), including:
- Down syndrome
- Papillon-Lefèvre syndrome
- Ehlers-Danlos syndrome
- hypophosphatasia
- Cohen syndrome
- Job syndrome
- glycogen storage disease.

Conditions which all have a genetic component but come under other categories:
- Infantile genetic agranulocytosis (haematological risk factor)
- Chédiak-Higashi syndrome (haematological risk factor)
- chronic granulomatous disease (haematological risk factor)
- type 1 diabetes (metabolic risk factor).

B. Environmental risk factors, e.g. drug therapies (see Box 3-1).

C. Behavioural risk factors, e.g. smoking (Box 3-2), poor oral hygiene compliance.

D. Life style risk factors, e.g. stress. This may be caused by major life events or daily minor hassles (LeResche and Dworkin 2002). Periodontal disease may result because stress:
- modulates neuroendocrine system
- depresses immune system
- increases the risk of inflammatory periodontal disease
- produces indirect behavioural effects which can lead to decreased oral hygiene, increased smoking, and risk of periodontal disease.

E. Metabolic risk factors, e.g. poorly controlled diabetes mellitus (see Box 3-3).

Box 3-1

Environmental Risk Factor: Drug Therapies
Nature of risk factor

- Drug-induced gingival overgrowth (DIGO) may occur as a side effect of three drug groups:

- Phenytoin (incidence, 50%), used to manage epilepsy

- Ciclosporin (incidence, 30%), used as an immunosuppressant after organ transplant or in severe psoriasis

- Calcium channel blocking drugs, used to manage hypertension, e.g. nifedepine, amlodipine, felodipine, etc. (incidence, 10–20%)

- DIGO involves the epithelial and connective tissues with excessive production of extracellular matrix, hence the terms hyperplasia or hypertrophy are no longer used

- Pathobiology of DIGO is highly complex, poorly understood and beyond the scope of this text (Seymour, et al. 2000)

Periodontal effects

- May develop within three months of starting drug

- Has predilection for anterior gingiva

- Has an increased propensity in children and adolescents that may relate to drug-related increases in gingival fibroblast androgen metabolism that targets subpopulations of fibroblasts that lead to elevated synthesis or a fall in collagenase activity

- Risk factors include age, gender, drug variables, concomitant medication, periodontal variables, genetic factors

- ↓ Inflammation with improved oral hygiene will facilitate surgical management

- May ↓ or resolve by ↓ drug dose or changing drug, e.g. replacing ciclosporin with tacrolimus in consultation with medical consultant and team

---

49

Box 3-2

Behavioural Risk Factor: Tobacco Smoking

Nature of risk factor

- Smoking habit often develops in adolescence – very few take up the habit after 18 years of age
- National and international surveys have shown that 14.4% of boys and girls smoke daily (Charlton 1996)
- Obtaining an accurate smoking history can be difficult for a young adult and even harder for an adolescent if the habit is hidden from accompanying adults; therefore make discreet enquiries, especially if nicotine staining or the characteristic odour of recent tobacco smoke is evident
- Numbers (n) of cigarettes smoked may be low at first
  - effects are cumulative
  - there is a dose-response relationship based on pack years (n of packs smoked/day x n of years smoked).
- Smokers aged 19–30 years 3.8 times more likely to have periodontitis than non-smoker and 51% of periodontitis attributable to smoking (Haber et al. 1993)
- Dental team should try to identify young smokers and aid in smoking cessation

Periodontal effects

Local and systemic effects on host defences:

- Inhibition of phagocytosis by polymorphonuclear leucocytes (PMNLs)
- ↓ Chemotaxis, migration of PMNLs
- Nicotine inhibits defensive functions of PMNLs, monocytes (↓ production of superoxide, IL-1β)
- ↓ Antibody production of serum IgG$_2$
- Altered peripheral immunoregulatory T-cell subset ratios
- ↓ Bone mineralisation
- ↓ Fibroblast function
- Adverse effect on microcirculation, gingival circulation, blood flow, chronic hypoxia of periodontal tissues (↓ bleeding and redness; pale, fibrotic gingiva)

Microbiological effects:

- Higher % of smokers than non-smokers are infected by B. forsythus, A. actinomycetemcomitans, P. gingivalis

Clinical periodontal effects in smokers:

- Greater prevalence, extent and severity of attachment loss, bone loss and pockets compared with similar age non-smokers with similar plaque levels
- Smokers respond less well to periodontal therapy
- Over 90% of refractory patients are smokers

Box 3-3

Metabolic Risk Factor: Poorly Controlled Diabetes

Nature of risk factor

- *Type 1 diabetes is most likely form of diabetes to present in children, adolescents and young adults*
- *Associated with destruction of pancreatic β cells; autoimmune process; specific genes identified (HLA-DR3, HLA-DR4)*
- *Onset is often abrupt*
- *Management involves daily insulin injections carefully balanced with carbohydrate intake*
- *Diabetes control can be problematic in children and in adolescents, the phenomena of insulin resistance and "teenage rebellion" exacerbate the situation*
- *Poorly controlled diabetes (measured by glycated haemoglobin (HbA_1C)) → hyperglycaemia*
- *Increased risk of diabetes complications with increased HbA_1C*
- *Increased severity of periodontal disease with increased HbA_1C*
- *Liase with diabetes care team re HbA_1C*

Periodontal effects link to:

- *Decreased PMNL function (chemotaxis, adherence, phagocytosis)*
- *Exaggerated inflammatory response (increased TNF-α, IL-1β, PGE_2)*
- *Decreased synthesis of collagen, glycosaminoglycan*
- *Increased collagenase*
- *Decreased production of bone matrix*
- *Collagen undergoes non-enzymatic glycation to advanced glycation end products (AGEs)*
- *AGEs increase cross-linking of collagen, decrease collagen solubility and turnover, stimulate hyper-responsive macrophages and lead to tissue destruction*

Clinical periodontal features relate to:

- *Severe attachment loss, bone loss and pockets*

F. Haematological risk factors (see Chapters 2, 6 and 7 for further details):
- infantile genetic agranulocytosis
- leucocyte adhesion deficiency (LAD)
- lazy leucocyte syndrome
- Chédiak-Higashi syndrome
- agamma/hypogammaglobulinaemia
- chronic granulomatous disease
- histiocytosis-X
- neutropenia
- lymphocyte deficiencies
- acute myeloblastic/lymphoblastic leukaemia
- acatalasia
- aplastic anaemia.

Comments about medical history
Genetic and haematological systemic periodontal risk factors are associated with non-plaque-induced gingival and periodontal conditions. These factors are discussed in Chapters 2, 6 and 7. Some conditions may be included in more than one category. For example, there is a genetic predisposition to Type 1 diabetes mellitus (HLA-DR3 and HLA-DR4 genes have been specifically linked) but since the periodontal effects principally relate to poor diabetes control, it has been included in the metabolic risk factors (Box 3-3).

Since an accurate medical history is required, details provided by the young adult, the adolescent or the child and parent or guardian may need to be supplemented with information from the general medical practitioner or consultant physician responsible for the patient's medical management before proceeding with the periodontal examination. Any systemic risk factor for periodontal disease identified during the history should be clearly recorded in the patient's clinical records.

Dental History
Information about past dental experiences indicates the nature and extent of treatment that the patient has undergone and how they coped with it. It is helpful to know whether the patient has had treatment provided under local analgesia, and if so, whether any particular problems or anxiety occurred.

Younger patients will often have had a limited range of dental experience and it is important to know prior to providing treatment if this is to be their first encounter a particular procedure. Sensitive questioning is required as going through an extensive list of treatments that a patient has not experienced (and perhaps never will), may be counterproductive and possibly provoke anxiety. Both the patient or guardian and their attitude to dental health and treatment will be relevant to the patient's management. Although this cannot necessarily be assessed at the first visit, information should be obtained on past dental experience and home oral care practices, which will give some insight into the dental awareness of the family. As the views of the patient and parent or guardian may not be the same, it may be worth addressing some questions to both.

Social History

In addition to the basic personal details that should be held on record for each patient (including name, address, date of birth), it is worth finding out if there is a preferred name or in the case of a child, a nickname, by which he/she prefers to be known. Other details that may be helpful in developing a rapport with the child include:

- the school attended
- which year they are in
- hobbies or interests
- the number of siblings and if siblings are older or younger than the patient.

The social background may have relevance as it might impact on the preventive measures that are feasible – parental occupation can be an indicator of this. For the older teenager and young adult, it is worth enquiring about availability to attend and preferred appointment times to minimise problems of missing college or time off work, etc. For parents bringing younger children, it is clearly essential to arrange times convenient to their work, home care or child care arrangements.

Enquiries can be made regarding oral hygiene routines, including:

- brushing frequency
- type of brush (manual or powered)
- type of dentifrice
- use of mouthwash
- nature and frequency and ease of use of any interdental cleaning aids, including floss, tape, interdental brush and single tufted interspace brush.

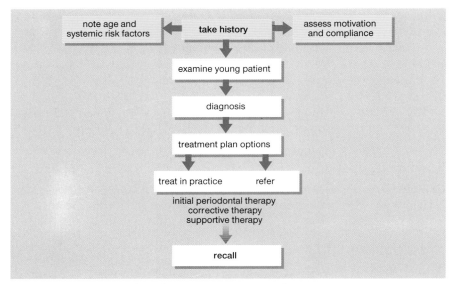

Fig 3-2 Stages in periodontal patient management: history.

History as an Aid to Diagnosis

The information elicited during the periodontal history, including identification of systemic risk factors for periodontal disease, needs to be interpreted along with the key findings from the dental and periodontal examination (Chapter 4) before reaching a diagnosis (Chapter 5) and formulating the treatment plan (Fig 3-2 and Chapter 8).

Key Points

- The history taking for a young patient or young adult presenting for a periodontal assessment should be structured and include relevant enquiries about:
  - presenting complaint, its history and reason for attendance
  - family history of periodontal problems and early tooth loss
  - previous medical history
  - previous dental history
  - social history.
- The medical history permits identification of patients of all ages who may:

- be predisposed to periodontal diseases
- pose a risk to the dental professional and other patients
- have systemic risk factors for periodontal diseases.
- Consent issues need to be addressed before proceeding with the subsequent periodontal examination and care of children, adolescents and young adults.
- The periodontal history together with the subsequent dental and periodontal examination provides a basis for the periodontal diagnosis.

References

Chapple ILC, Gilbert AD. Understanding Periodontal Diseases: Assessment and Diagnostic Procedures in Practice. London: Quintessence, 2002:99–146.

Charlton A. Children and smoking: the family circle. In: Doll R, Crofton J (Eds.) Tobacco and Health. RSM Press, Br Med Bulletin 1996;52:90–107.

Haber J, Wattles J, Crowley M, et al. Evidence for cigarette smoking as a major risk factor for periodontitis. J Periodontol 1993;64:16–23.

LeResche L, Dworkin SF. The role of stress in inflammatory disease, including periodontal disease: review of concepts and current findings. Periodontol 2000. 2002;29:91–103.

Seymour RA, Ellis JS, Thomason JM. Risk factors for drug-induced gingival overgrowth. J Clin Periodontol 2000;27:217–223.

Further Reading

American Academy of Periodontology. Diabetes and periodontal diseases. Position paper. J Periodontol 1999;70:935–949.

American Academy of Periodontology. Tobacco use and the periodontal patient. Position paper. J Periodontol 1999;70:1419–1427.

Department of Health. Reference guide to consent for examination or treatment. Website: www.doh.gov.uk./consent. 2001.

Chapter 4

Clinical Examination and Local Risk Factors for Periodontal Diseases

Aims

This chapter outlines the key stages of the initial periodontal examination for children, adolescents and young adults and describes local risk factors for the periodontal diseases relevant to this age group.

Outcome

Having read this chapter, the practitioner should understand the key stages of the periodontal examination of children, adolescents and young adults and be able to identify local periodontal risk factors pertinent to these patients. They should also appreciate the role of the Basic Periodontal Examination (BPE) in screening young adults and be familiar with the use of a simplified form of the BPE for children and adolescents. In addition, the reader will also be familiar with current regulations and guidance for the use of radiographs in young patients with periodontal diseases.

Examining Children, Adolescents and Young Adults

The routine dental examination (Fig 4-1a) of children, adolescents and young adults should include the following:
- Extraoral examination
- Intraoral examination (Fig 4-1b):
  - soft tissue examination
  - dental charting of teeth present, restorations, cavities, etc.
  - general description of periodontal condition, to include:
    - ❏ gingival colour
    - ❏ gingival contour
    - ❏ presence of swelling
    - ❏ presence and location of inflammation
    - ❏ presence of gingival recession
    - ❏ presence of suppuration
    - ❏ qualitative assessment of oral hygiene and presence of supragingival calculus deposits

❏ occlusal problems, drifting/tooth migration and related aesthetic problems.
– identification of local periodontal risk factors
– screening using BPE
– special tests:
  ❏ radiographs
  ❏ vitality tests.

The general principles and details of the examination are described in the first book of this series (see Chapple and Gilbert 2002), therefore the present account will focus on the key aspects of local factors, screening and radiographs that pertain to the younger age groups.

Local Risk Factors

Local risk factors can increase the risk of periodontal disease development and progression principally by acting as plaque retention factors. These factors should be investigated during a thorough dental examination of the patient (Box 4-1).

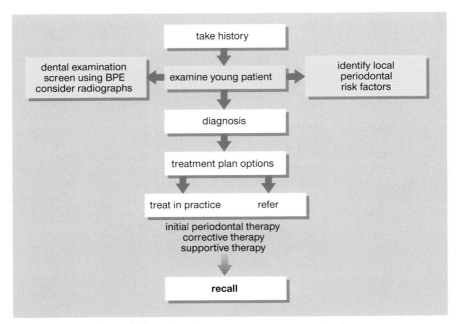

Fig 4-1a Stages in periodontal patient management: examination.

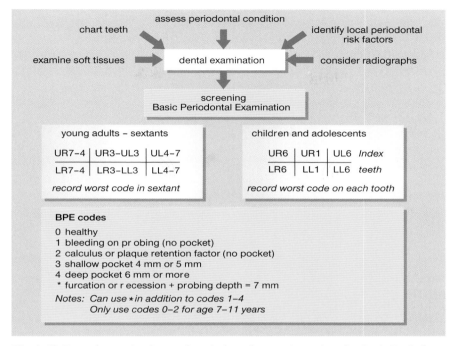

Fig 4-1b Dental examination and periodontal screening using the Basic Periodontal Examination (BPE) for children, adolescents and young adults.

Box 4-1

Local Risk Factors for Periodontal Diseases

- *Calculus (supra- and subgingival)*
- *Restorations*
- *Fraenal attachments*
- *Orthodontic appliances*
- *Malocclusion or crowding/imbrication*
- *Local trauma*
- *Mouth breathing and lack of lip seal*
- *Xerostomia*
- *Anatomical features*

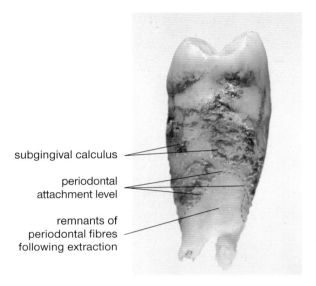

subgingival calculus

periodontal
attachment level

remnants of
periodontal fibres
following extraction

Fig 4-2 Subgingival calculus in association with loss of attachment on extracted tooth.

Calculus

Supra- and subgingival calculus deposits act as local plaque retention factors. Although calculus deposits are expected in adults, subgingival calculus is also common in teenagers. It has been shown that subgingival calculus is related to gingival inflammation and attachment loss in adolescents (Fig 4-2). A relationship has also been found between ethnicity and subgingival calculus deposits in adolescents with deposits more prevalent in young Asian patients.

Restorations

Subgingival restoration margins, marginal discrepancies and overhanging restorations have all been associated with gingivitis and attachment loss due to the difficulties they present for plaque removal – not for direct irritation of the tissues. In Western countries there has been a trend towards improved child dental health over the past decade. With further caries prevention measures, there should be fewer restorations impacting on the gingival tissues. Nevertheless, dental caries is still a common condition, particularly in areas of social deprivation. Sites with extensive proximal caries have been associated with bone loss and restoration of such sites has been associated with bony infill. The use of matrix bands, wedges, the adaptation of stainless steel crown margins and careful clinical and laboratory techniques for the provision of cast restorations will help to produce restorations in the young patient that should not have any future periodontal consequences.

Fraenal Attachment

A prominent fraenum can act as a local plaque retention factor by impeding access to the toothbrush (Fig 4-3a and b). Direct fraenal pull has been described as an aetiological factor in gingival recession, but this is unlikely to be a common contributing factor.

Orthodontic Appliances

Fixed and removable orthodontic appliances are commonly worn by children and adolescents and considerable effort is required by the patient to maintain a clean mouth (Fig 4-4). Some young adults wear orthodontic appliances for the alignment of teeth that have drifted due to periodontal disease once the disease has stabilised following periodontal therapy. Important issues to consider include:

- access to interdental cleaning is diminished and plaque is more likely to accumulate
- gingivitis commonly occurs after placement of fixed orthodontic appliances and enamel decalcification can occur around bonded attachments

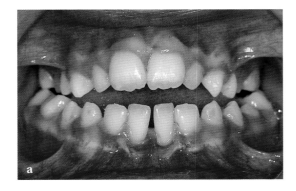

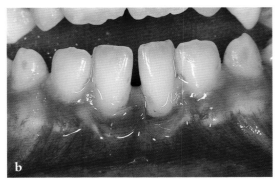

Fig 4-3 (a,b) High fraenal attachments impeding tooth brushing. (b) Note plaque deposits in association with localised gingival recession in 11-year-girl.

- teeth with bands are harder to access for cleaning and bands extending to the gingival tissues increase the likelihood of plaque retention and gingivitis
- if oral hygiene is good then the deleterious effects are minimal
- coronal attachment loss can occur during orthodontic appliance therapy and can range from an annual loss of 0.05–0.3mm
- apical root resorption is also a common consequence of orthodontic treatment that results in a reduced length of root (Fig 4-5) supported by bone even though no coronal (plaque-induced) alveolar bone loss has occurred in these circumstances
- direct trauma from components of orthodontic appliances can cause local injury to the soft tissues
- chronic trauma may lead to gingival overgrowth or a fibrous epulis may develop (Fig 4-6)
- if teeth are orthodontically moved within alveolar bone there is generally little risk of soft tissue recession
- orthodontic tooth movements associated with excessive proclination of lower incisors and arch expansion do carry an increased risk of gingival recession. It is important to anticipate this scenario and consider a pre-orthodontic connective tissue graft to provide a keratinised labial gingiva (Fig 4-7a,b)

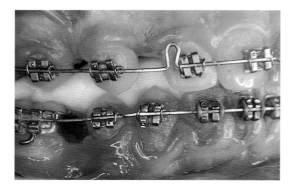

Fig 4-4 Plaque around fixed orthodontic appliance, disclosed in the lower arch to aid visibility.

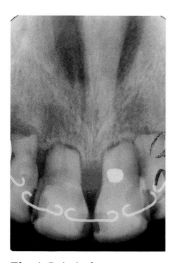

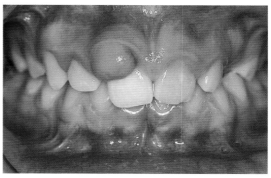

Fig 4-6 Fibrous epulis related to chronic irritation from subgingival calculus acting as a plaque retention factor.

Fig 4-5 Apical root resorption following orthodontic treatment.

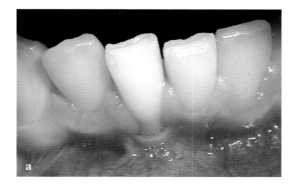

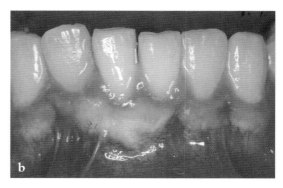

Fig 4-7 (a,b) Pre-orthodontic connective tissue graft to provide keratinised labial gingiva; (a) pre-graft, (b) post-graft surgery.

Malocclusion

An association between irregularity of teeth and gingivitis has been demonstrated. Oral hygiene measures are harder to implement at sites where teeth are imbricated, rotated, markedly retroclined or proclined. However a lack of orthodontic treatment does not seem to have much effect on periodontal diseases later in life. A severe overbite can cause direct trauma to the upper palatal or lower labial gingival tissues which may be associated with gingival recession.

Local Trauma

Direct local trauma can be the result of habits such as an aggressive tooth brushing technique or factitious injury from fingernail picking at the gingival margin (Fig 4-8a,b). These habits may lead to gingival recession, attachment loss and bone loss (Figure 4-8c).

Mouth Breathing and Lack of Lip Seal

Mouth breathing, lack of lip coverage at rest and lack of lip seal (incompetent lips) are associated with higher levels of plaque and gingivitis, all of which are not infrequent in the developing child and adolescent (Fig 4-9). It appears that mouth breathing is related to gingivitis of the maxillary anterior teeth while lip coverage influences gingivitis on labial and palatal surfaces.

Xerostomia

Xerostomia is a side effect of radiotherapy with radiation fields including the salivary glands. In children the management of nasopharyngeal carcinomas and rhabdomyosarcomas of the orbit may produce xerostomia. Some types of chemotherapy can produce xerostomia, but this is usually transient. Xerostomia can be associated with increased gingivitis due to lack of the innate defensive functions of saliva. It may also be a feature in HIV-positive children.

Anatomical Features

Enamel projections and pearls (Fig 4-10), proximal and palatogingival grooves (Fig 4-11) are all developmental dental features and have been associated with gingivitis and attachment loss. Cemental tears are defined as complete separation of the cement from the dentine or partial separation within the cement layer and these may be associated with attachment loss. The prevalence of these tears in the young has not been documented.

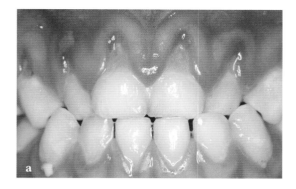

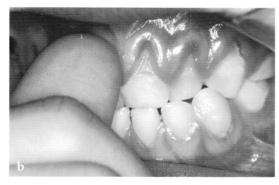

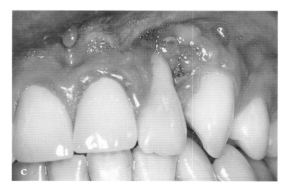

Fig 4-8 (a,b) Gingival recession resulting from fingernail picking at gingival margin. (c) Loss of attachment and bone loss as a consequence of the habit.

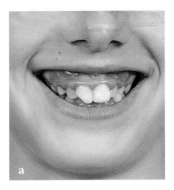
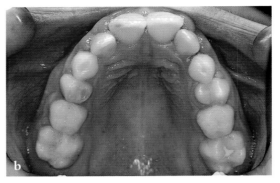

Fig 4-9 (a) Twelve-year-old boy who breathes through his mouth, with high lip line and lack of lip seal (incompetent lips). (b) Due to lack of protective effects of saliva the gingivitis is more pronounced on the labial aspect of the anteriors than palatally or posteriorly

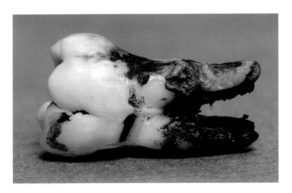

Fig 4-10 Enamel projection into bifurcation in association with buccal attachment loss on stained extracted mandibular molar.

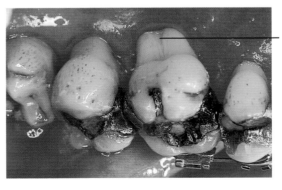

root groove

Fig 4-11 Palatal root groove.

66

Periodontal Screening

Since the recommendation of the British Society of Periodontology in 1986 to introduce periodontal screening into general dental practice using the Community Periodontal Index of Treatment Needs (CPITN), the index has been reconfigured as the Basic Periodontal Examination. The BPE provides a quick and simple method of screening all patients for periodontal problems. It is comfortably tolerated and gives the practitioner an indication of the need for periodontal treatment and the level of further periodontal examination required for differing periodontal disease levels.

The BPE is not intended as a replacement for periodontal indices designed to measure "periodontal status", such as the six-point per tooth measurement of probing pocket depths (Chapter 8). It is intended to determine which patients will benefit from a more detailed periodontal examination and may require more complex periodontal therapy. It assesses and codes for the presence of bleeding, calculus or plaque retention factors, and pockets (see Fig 4-1b). However, it does not record plaque levels or details of attachment loss and recession.

Using the BPE in Children, Adolescents and Young Adults

WHO 621 Probe

The BPE is performed using the WHO 621 probe (Fig 4-12) that has a 0.5mm spherical ball on the tip and black band at 3.5–5.5mm to delineate normal sulci (<3.5mm) and periodontal pockets (>3.5mm). The ball end on this probe is very useful for detecting subgingival calculus deposits. This procedure can be comfortably undertaken on young individuals provided the recommended probing force of 20–25g (0.20–0.25N) is not exceeded. Additional marks at 8.5mm and 11.5mm are present on the WHO "C-type" probe version for clinical use (Fig 4-12).

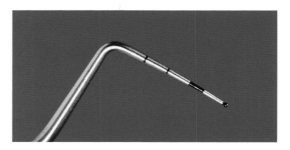

Fig 4-12 WHO 621-C version probe with 0.5mm ball tip, black band at 3.5–5.5mm and additional markings at 8.5mm and 11.5mm.

Sextants/Index Teeth

In young adults, the mouth is divided into sextants as depicted in Fig 4-1b. At least two teeth must be present in a sextant for it to be scored, otherwise the single tooth should be included in the score for the neighbouring sextant. In teenagers and children, following full eruption of the incisors and first permanent molars, screening using the BPE can be undertaken on the index teeth UR6, UR1, UL6, LL6, LL1 and LR6.

Recording BPE

In young adults, the probe should be gently walked around all the teeth in each sextant, whereas in children and teenagers the probe is gently walked around each index tooth, covering six sites per tooth:

- distobuccal
- buccal
- mesiobuccal
- distolingual
- lingual
- mesiolingual.

The worst finding in each sextant or for each index tooth is recorded using a six box grid, and the codes 0, 1, 2, 3, 4, ★ (Figs 4-13 and 4-14). This should only take a minute or so in young adults, and even less time in children and teenagers.

It is recommended that only codes 0, 1, 2 should be determined up to the age of 11 years because of the likelihood of false pockets associated with newly erupting teeth. However, if the black band on the WHO 621 probe disappears into any unusually deep pockets, then further periodontal investigation is required, irrespective of age. In adolescents, the full range of scores can be used on the index teeth so that periodontal pockets can be detected as early as possible, although care should be exercised to distinguish true pockets with attachment loss (Fig 4-15) from false pockets (see Fig 1-12). Other periodontal indices (described in Chapter 8) will need to be recorded depending on the BPE codes (Fig 4-16). If pockets are detected, then full mouth periodontal indices (Fig 4-16) and subsequent monitoring should be undertaken (see Chapter 8) and the need for radiographs considered (see below).

Frequency of Recording BPE

While guidelines on the frequency of undertaking periodontal screening have been proposed for adults by the British Society of Periodontology (Box 4-2), these are generally lacking for younger age groups. Since screening of six index

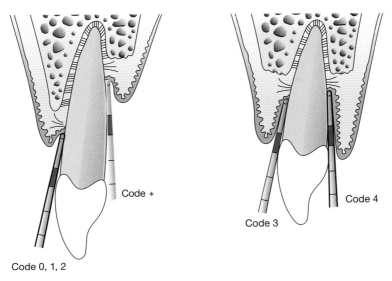

Code *

Code 0, 1, 2

Code 3

Code 4

Fig 4-13 Basic Periodontal Examination codes 0,1, 2 and ★.

Fig 4-14 Basic Periodontal Examination codes 3 and 4.

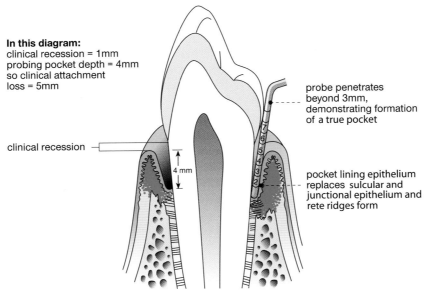

In this diagram:
clinical recession = 1mm
probing pocket depth = 4mm
so clinical attachment
loss = 5mm

clinical recession

4 mm

probe penetrates
beyond 3mm,
demonstrating formation
of a true pocket

pocket lining epithelium
replaces sulcular and
junctional epithelium and
rete ridges form

Fig 4-15 Schematic longitudinal section of a premolar and associated periodontal tissues, demonstrating early true pocket formation detected by clinical probing.

69

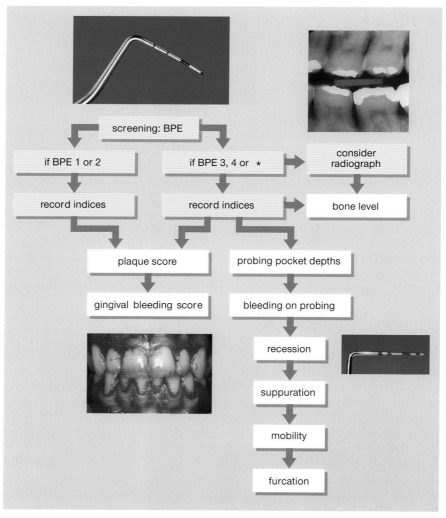

Fig 4-16 Schematic of the other periodontal indices required for the various Basic Periodontal Examination codes.

70

teeth is very quick, simple and acceptable to young patients, it seems prudent to recommend periodontal screening of all new child or adolescent patients and this should be repeated following the principles outlined in Box 4-2.

Box 4-2

Frequency of Recording BPE

- *All new patients*
- *Patient requiring advanced restorative treatment or orthodontic treatment*
- *If BPE = 0, screen again within one year*
- *If BPE = 1 or 2, treat and screen within one year*
- *If BPE = 3 in one or more sextants, treat and review. If still code 3, record full periodontal indices in affected sextants (see Chapter 8 for details of indices)*
- *If BPE = 4 or ★, record full periodontal indices and consider referral*

Use of Radiographs

In the UK, dentists must comply with the legal requirements of the:
- Ionising Radiation Regulations 1999 (IRR99).
- Ionising Radiation (Medical Exposures) Regulations 2000 (IR(ME)R2000).

IRR99 regulations relate mainly to the protection of workers and the public, and also address the equipment aspects of patient protection. IR(ME)R2000 regulations identify referrers, practitioners and operators and define the responsibilities of employers and clinicians. Guidance notes for dental practitioners are available that summarise the measures that must be taken when using radiographic equipment to comply with the current regulations (National Radiological Protection Board, 2001). Although the principles of these regulations can be considered good practice for the use of radiographs, details of the legislation in force outside the UK will vary from country to country.

Justification
Justification of the medical exposure should be based on the practitioner's knowledge of the hazards associated with the exposure and on the relevant clinical information. The UK regulations emphasise that it is illegal to carry

out a radiographic exposure of a patient without a good clinical indication and unless the radiograph may change patient management, and furthermore, that those responsible for justification of the radiograph may be deemed to be criminally liable.

Optimisation

Optimisation is the means by which radiation doses arising from exposures are kept as low as is reasonably achievable and it is also a requirement of the radiation regulations. The following measures can be applied to minimise radiation dose:

- Intraoral films used should be E-speed or faster.
- Beam should be collimated by use of a rectangular collimator.
- Intraoral equipment should be fitted with a long cone (>200mm).
- Film holders should be used for bitewing and periapical radiography.
- Paralleling technique for periapical radiographs should be used.
- Intensifying screens should be used in panoramic radiography to reduce dosage.

It is anticipated that the uptake of digital radiography in general practice is set to increase over the next few years, replacing the need for film altogether. The radiation dose is lower than for film in a number of digital systems.

In children, it is especially important that the radiation dosage be kept as low as possible. The tissues of younger people are more radiosensitive than those of adults. Children are at greater risk of cancer from x-ray exposure than adults because the child's prospective lifespan is likely to exceed the latent period between the exposure and clinical presentation of a cancer. This is limited in contrast to an exposure in a patient of 80 years of age for whom the risk would be reduced.

A BPE code of 3, 4 or *, or a periodontal charting that has shown pocketing or furcation involvement will warrant radiographic examination if there are no recent films available.

Radiographic Information

Radiographs can provide the clinician with a large amount of information of periodontal significance:

- Degree and the pattern of bone loss:
  - horizontal bone loss – may indicate chronic periodontitis
  - vertical (infrabony) bone loss – may indicate aggressive disease or occlusal trauma

- if apex visible, the percentage bone loss is calculable against root length.
- Root morphology.
- Progression of bone loss using serial films.
- Position of the normal, healthy bony crest:
  - 0.4–1.9mm from the cemento-enamel junction (CEJ) around permanent teeth
  - may be greater than 2mm in deciduous teeth (unstable)
  - may also increase with facial growth and with the loss of an adjacent deciduous tooth or eruption of a neighbouring permanent tooth.
- Furcation defects.
- Subgingival calculus deposits (associated with attachment loss and bone loss in adolescents).
- Overhanging restoration margins and caries.
- Apical pathology.
- Other pathology, e.g. retained root, cyst, supernumerary teeth, odontomes, etc.

Radiographic Views

The radiographic view selected should be determined by the diagnostic information required. Several views can be utilised:
- horizontal bitewing
- vertical bitewing
- periapical
- panoramic.

Horizontal bitewing radiographs are recommended for the detection of caries with frequency dependent on caries risk. These radiographs can be very useful in assessing a patient for periodontal disease. The alveolar crest is imaged on bitewing radiographs even if there has been some degree of bone loss. A consistent geometry can be achieved which enables useful longitudinal monitoring of bone changes (Fig 4-17).

Vertical bitewing radiographs are taken by rotating the conventional intraoral film through 90° so that the longer length of the film is vertically positioned. This results in a radiograph which shows a more extensive bone image and can still image several teeth on each film (Fig 4-18).

Periapical radiographs taken at selected sites can be used where information on the apical status is needed in addition to bone levels and bone morphology. These should be taken using a long cone paralleling technique that will

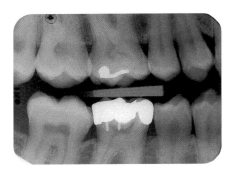

Fig 4-17 Horizontal bitewing radiograph.

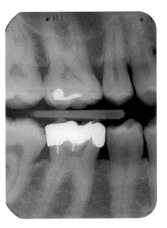

Fig 4-18 Vertical bitewing radiograph.

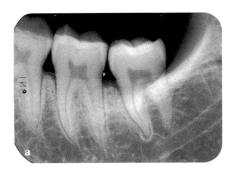

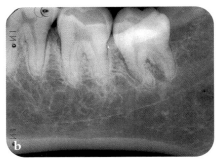

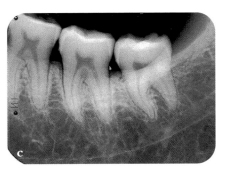

Fig 4-19 (a–c) Periapical radiographs; (a) elongated by bisecting angle, (b) foreshortened by bisecting angle, (c) paralleling technique used to provide correct angulation. Note "apparent" differences in bone loss LL6-7 interdental space.

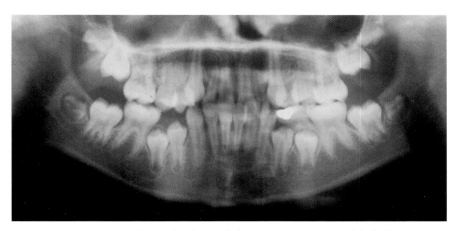

Fig 4-20 Panoramic radiograph of mixed dentition in 10-year-old child.

enable a consistent image to be taken. Although the bisected angle technique is still used by some dentists for periapical radiography, it is unsuitable, in particular, for the periodontal assessment of patients. There is an inherent tendency in the bisected angle technique for bone loss to be underestimated because of the angulation of the beam in relation to the film (Fig 4-19a–c). Panoramic radiographs may be indicated for orthodontic treatment planning to determine the presence or absence of permanent teeth and the location of unerupted teeth. Such radiographs may be well tolerated in the younger patient (Fig 4-20). Bone levels can be determined from panoramic radiographs although these radiographs suffer from the disadvantages of overlap of teeth and reduced image quality in the anterior regions. However, selected periapical radiographs can be taken to supplement the panoramic radiograph once the latter has been reviewed.

Radiographic Report

The opportunity to assess bone levels on intraoral or panoramic films should always be taken, whether or not these were taken primarily for periodontal purposes. Even in the absence of any clinical findings, radiographs should be read to confirm that there is no periodontal disease. It is not uncommon for radiographic signs of periodontal disease to be overlooked simply because the disease was not expected and therefore not looked for on the radiographs. Legislation in the UK requires the dentist to produce a report of radiographic findings. This need not be a lengthy account, but an entry in the patient's notes should indicate that films have been assessed for signs of disease and pertinent findings recorded (Box 4-3).

Box 4-3

Example of Brief Radiographic Report

Radiographs show:

Maxilla — *bone loss generalised (~20–30%) and largely horizontal. Vertical defect UL6 mesially (~70%) and bone loss UR7 (50%).*

Mandible — *crestal bone loss only LR molars. Lower anteriors 40% horizontal bone loss, funnel defect LL4 (? occlusal trauma) and 10–20% bone loss LL molars.*

UR1 has perio-endo lesion and UR7 recurrent caries under distal restoration.

Guidelines

The radiation regulations require the "referrers" to have access to guidelines or referral criteria for radiographs. In 1998 the Faculty of General Dental Practitioners (UK) published *Selection criteria for dental radiography* - a very useful document for dentists working in primary dental care.

Key Points

- The periodontal examination of the young patient should be structured to include:
  - Extraoral examination.
  - Intraoral examination:
    - ❏ soft tissue examination
    - ❏ dental chart
    - ❏ general description of periodontal condition
    - ❏ identification of local periodontal risk factors
    - ❏ screening using BPE
    - ❏ special tests, such as radiographs.
- Local risk factors for periodontal diseases need to be identified during the periodontal examination of the young person.
- Periodontal screening should be undertaken for the young adult using the BPE; a simplified form of the BPE may be used for the adolescent or child.
- Valuable information can be gleaned from radiographs; each radiograph must be clinically justified and reported on in the notes.

References

Chapple ILC, Gilbert AD. Understanding Periodontal Diseases: Assessment and Diagnostic Procedures in Practice. London: Quintessence, 2002:99–146.

Faculty of General Dental Practitioners (UK). Selection criteria for dental radiography. London: FGDP, 1998.

National Radiological Protection Board. Guidance notes for dental practitioners on the safe use of x-ray equipment. London: National Radiological Protection Board and Department of Health, 2001.

Chapter 5
Periodontal Diagnosis in Young Patients

Aim

The aim of this chapter is to outline the principles of diagnosis and key features of periodontal conditions that the dental practitioner may come across when caring for children, adolescents and young adults.

Outcomes

Most of the periodontal problems that the young patient may experience are plaque-induced, but some uncommon conditions are not. After reading this chapter, the practitioner should understand how to reach a periodontal diagnosis in the young patient and should be able to diagnose the principal periodontal diseases that can affect children, adolescents and young adults. The reader will also understand how important systemic risk factors such as smoking, poorly controlled diabetes or stress can influence the presentation of periodontal diseases in the young.

Principles of Periodontal Diagnosis

A periodontal diagnosis is reached after consideration of findings from the history (Chapter 3) and examination (Chapter 4) and requires an awareness of the current classification of periodontal diseases as discussed in Chapter 1 (Fig 5-1).

Based on the current classification system of the 1999 International Workshop, the diagnosis should fall within one of the main classification categories or its subdivisions (see Table 1-1):
A. Dental plaque-induced gingival diseases.
B. Non-plaque-induced gingival lesions.
C. Chronic periodontitis.
D. Aggressive periodontitis.
E. Periodontitis as a manifestation of systemic disease.
F. Necrotising periodontal diseases.
G. Abscesses of the periodontium.
H. Periodontitis associated with endodontic lesions.
I. Developmental or acquired deformities and conditions.

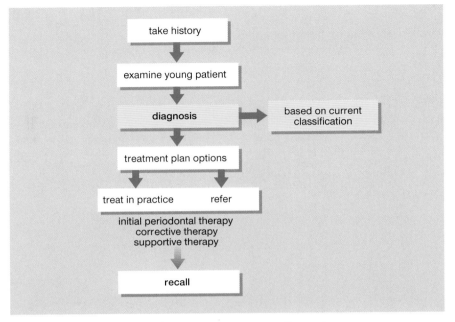

Fig 5-1 Stages in periodontal patient management: diagnosis.

This chapter will cover the key clinical and radiographic diagnostic features of the principal periodontal diseases in categories A, C, D and F – I that affect children, adolescents and young adults. Category B is covered in Chapter 6 and category E is covered in Chapter 7.

Gingival Diseases

The most common form of gingivitis is dental plaque-induced gingivitis, with key diagnostic features are shown in Box 5-1. This may present with or without local risk factors such as supra- and subgingival calculus (Fig 5-2) or mouth breathing (Fig 5-3).

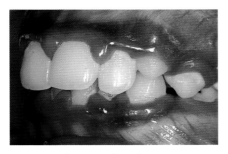

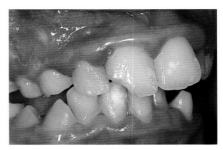

Fig 5-2 Plaque-induced gingivitis in a 10-year-old Asian girl. Supragingival calculus visible at buccal margins of LL1, LL2 and erupting UL4.

Fig 5-3 A twelve-year-old who breathes through his mouth, with lack of lip seal (incompetent lips). Note the gingiva is more inflamed anteriorly than posteriorly due to lack of the protective effects of saliva.

Box 5-1

Diagnostic Features of Plaque-induced Gingivitis

- *Plaque present at gingival margin*

- *Change in gingival colour, contour*

- *Increased gingival crevicular fluid (GCF) from sulcus, and increased sulcular temperature*

- *Bleeding from margin of gingiva on provocation, e.g. probing*

- *No attachment loss*

- *No bone loss*

- *Basic Periodontal Examination (BPE) = 1 and/or BPE = 2 are compatible with diagnosis of gingivitis*

- *False gingival pockets ≥4mm may be present due to gingival swelling*

- *False pockets should be distinguished from true periodontal pockets ≥4mm*

- *Clinical and histological changes are reversible on removal of plaque*

- *Plaque-induced gingivitis can develop on a reduced periodontium following resolution of previous periodontitis where pre-existing attachment loss or bone loss may be present*

Other forms of plaque-induced gingivitis include those associated with systemic risk factors, e.g. pregnancy (Fig 5-4) or drug-induced gingival overgrowth (Fig 5-5a,b).

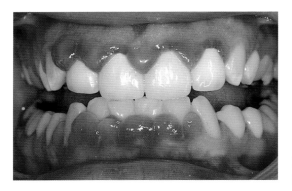

Fig 5-4 Pregnancy-related gingivitis in a young patient.

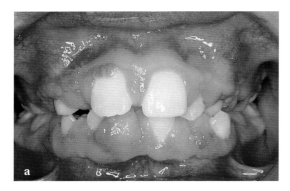

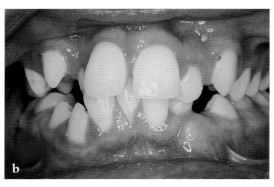

Fig 5-5 (a) Drug-induced gingival overgrowth in a teenage boy taking ciclosporin and nifedipine following a heart transplant. (b) Drug-induced gingival overgrowth reduced when the two drugs were replaced with tacrolimus and a non-calcium-channel blocking drug.

Chronic Periodontitis

Incipient Chronic Periodontitis

Since the transition from reversible gingivitis to incipient chronic periodontitis can affect a sizeable proportion of teenagers (Chapter 1), Basic Periodontal Examination (BPE) screening should be undertaken at the initial consultation in this age group and at recall visits (Box 5-2, Fig 5-6). Radiographs should be reviewed for bone loss, especially if serial views of intraoral films are available. Horizontal bitewings are particularly useful for assessing crestal bone levels in this age group.

If there is any doubt as to whether pockets are true or false, the presence of clinical loss of attachment should be determined. In this age group, the "one-stage technique" is useful for measuring small amounts of clinical loss of attachment (1–3mm): the cemento-enamel junction (CEJ) is located by tactile sensation and the distance advanced by the probe apically from this position is noted until the clinical attachment level (i.e. base of the pocket) is reached (Figs 5-7 and 5-8).

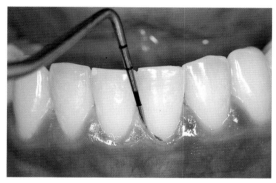

Fig 5-6 Basic Periodontal Examination screening of one of the index teeth in a 17-year-old Asian girl.

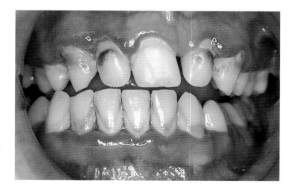

Fig 5-7 A 19-year-old patient with incipient chronic periodontitis.

83

Box 5-2

Diagnostic Features of Chronic Periodontitis

Incipient chronic periodontitis

- *Age of onset can be in adolescence (13–14 years)*
- *Interproximal clinical attachment loss of 1–2mm (commonly seen on maxillary first molars, mandibular incisors), associated with presence of plaque, subgingival calculus*
- *Pockets 4–5mm (screening BPE = 3)*
- *Bone loss no more than ~0.5mm over an 18-month period (bitewing radiographs typically show horizontal pattern of bone loss)*
- *If BPE = 4 or BPE = * in adolescence, suspect aggressive periodontitis (see below)*

Established chronic periodontitis

- *Presence of interproximal clinical loss of attachment (CAL)*
- *True pocket formation ≥4mm (screening by BPE = 3 or BPE = 4)*
- *Bone loss evident on radiographic examination, typically, horizontal pattern of bone loss although vertical bone loss may be present at some sites*
- *Possible (variable) presence of drifting, inflammation, mobility, recession and furcation defects (BPE = *)*
- *Slow to moderate progression and exacerbations*
- *Can be further classified according to extent of CAL (localised ≤30% sites affected; generalised >30% affected) and severity (slight = CAL 1–2mm; moderate = 3–4mm, severe ≥5mm)*
- *Plaque control inadequate; supragingival calculus frequent finding*
- *Variable subgingival plaque microbiota, e.g.* P. gingivalis, P. intermedia, A. actinomycetemcomitans
- *Destruction consistent with presence of local factors, e.g. subgingival calculus*
- *Modifying factors include local predisposing factors, poorly controlled diabetes, stress and smoking*

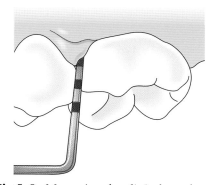 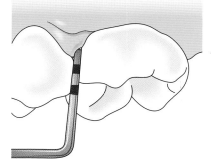

Fig 5-8a Measuring the clinical attachment level: periodontal probe tip located at CEJ on tooth. CEJ located by tactile sensation.

Fig 5-8b Measuring the clinical attachment level: periodontal probe tip located 1mm apical to CEJ at clinical attachment level, indicating loss of attachment of 1mm.

Chronic Periodontitis

With increasing age, the cumulative effects of attachment loss, pocket formation and alveolar bone loss progressively and slowly increase the prevalence, extent and severity of chronic periodontitis. Exacerbations can occur at times of stress, or resumption of a smoking habit.

Smoking-related Chronic Periodontitis

Young patients who smoke show more severe clinical attachment loss, pockets and radiographic bone loss than same-age peers with similar plaque levels as explained in earlier chapters (Chapters 1 and 3). Typical diagnostic features are the pale, fibrous gingiva, which have less tendency to bleed on probing due to the vasoconstrictive effects of tobacco components. Maxillary anterior and palatal surfaces are adversely affected and anterior recession may be a presenting feature. Nicotine staining is readily detectable and often increased supragingival calculus formation is seen. These features form the basis of a diagnosis of smoking-related chronic periodontitis (Fig 5-9). Smoking can just as readily influence the severity of the presentation of aggressive forms of periodontitis.

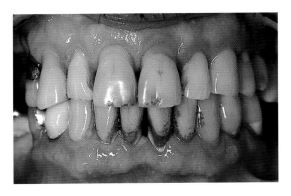

Fig 5-9 A lifetime's exposure to cigarette smoking beyond adolescence and young adulthood into middle age is associated with smoking-related chronic periodontitis. Note the pale fibrous gingivae, anterior recession, nicotine staining and supragingival calculus.

Aggressive Periodontitis

Because of the rapidly destructive nature of this condition, early diagnosis is especially important so that therapy can be instigated as soon as possible. There are two forms: localised and generalised.

Localised Aggressive Periodontitis

The localised form of aggressive periodontitis can present around puberty, and specifically affects first molars and incisors (unlike incipient chronic periodontitis that can affect these and other sites). The key diagnostic features are listed in Box 5-3. Unlike chronic periodontitis, phagocyte abnormalities can be present and there may be a hyperresponsive macrophage or neutrophil phenotype (see Chapter 1).

This is an excellent example of a periodontal disease where a specific microbial aetiology has been implicated. The micro-organism involved, *A. actinomycetemcomitans*, is a particularly virulent periodontal pathogen that possesses a number of strategies to try to evade the host's defence mechanisms. The progression of periodontal destruction in both the localised and the generalised forms may possibly be self-limiting in some individuals, however, this is unpredictable and the consequences irreversibly severe, and therefore early diagnosis should always be a priority (Figs 5-10–5-13).

Box 5-3

Diagnostic Features of Localised Aggressive Periodontitis

- *Onset around puberty*

- *Tendency to aggregate in families – check family history*

- *Patients are clinically healthy apart from presence of periodontitis*

- *Uncommon condition, but predilection for certain ethnic groups: Black (2.6%), Caucasian (0.1–0.2%)*

- *No gender predilection*

- *Localised first molar/incisor presentation*

- *Interproximal attachment loss >3mm on at least two permanent teeth, one of which is a first molar, and involving no more than two teeth other than the first molars/incisors*

- *BPE = 4, BPE = ★ during screening of adolescents – if present, check for interproximal attachment loss (as above)*

- *Plaque levels not always commensurate with amount of periodontal destruction*

- *Subgingival calculus may or may not be a significant feature*

- *Gingival inflammation may or may not be a significant feature*

- *Alveolar bone loss:*

  – arc shaped defects on first molars

  – vertical (infrabony) bone loss/angular defects on incisors

  – may be symmetrical right and left

  – may be incidental finding on bitewings for caries or panoramic radiograph for orthodontics

Important features of inflammatory – immune response

- *Robust serum antibody response to* A. actinomycetemcomitans

- *Phagocyte abnormalities in some individuals*

- *May have hyperresponsive macrophage/PMNL phenotype, including increased PGE_2 and IL-1β*

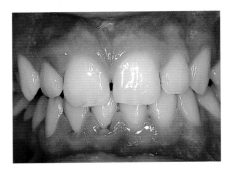

Fig 5-10 A 13-year-old boy with localised aggressive periodontitis: little clinical evidence of severe periodontal problems to the untrained eye.

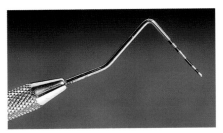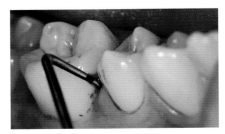

Fig 5-11 (a) PCP10 pocket measuring probe. (b) 8mm probing pocket depth – LR6.

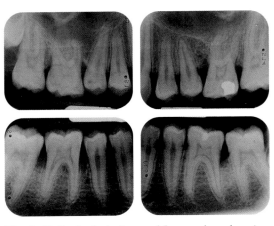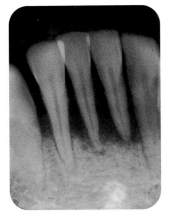

Fig 5-12 Periapical views of first molars showing typical arc-shaped bone loss in the patient shown in Figs 5-10 and 5-11. Relatively early diagnosis was made by the patient's general dental practitioner.

Fig 5-13 Periapical view of mandibular incisors in another 13-year-old boy who was diagnosed late as having localised aggressive periodontitis. Note the advanced bone loss and poor prognosis.

Generalised Aggressive Periodontitis

Generalised aggressive periodontitis can be quite difficult to diagnose and distinguish from a severe form of advanced chronic periodontitis – this is reflected in the changes in criteria in the various classifications over the years. The diagnostic features according to the current classification are summarised in Box 5-4. Any young adult under the age of 30 years presenting with BPE code = 4 or ★ in all (or most) sextants, needs to be considered as a potential case of generalised aggressive periodontitis (Fig 5-14 and Fig 5-15).

Box 5-4

Diagnostic Features of Generalised Aggressive Periodontitis

- *Age usually <30 years although may be older. Can affect adolescents*

- *Generalised interproximal clinical attachment loss >3mm on at least three teeth other than first molars and incisors*

- *Concomitant alveolar bone loss*

- *Generalised and severe horizontal bone loss*

- *Vertical bone loss may be evident and widespread*

- *Pronounced episodic nature of destruction of attachment and alveolar bone*

- *Patients clinically healthy apart from presence of periodontitis*

- *Plaque levels may not be commensurate with amount of periodontal destruction*

- *Presence of subgingival calculus associated with clinical attachment loss*

- *Gingival inflammation may or may not be evident*

Important features of inflammatory immune response

- *Poor serum antibody response to infecting agents* A. actinomycetemcomitans, P. gingivalis

- *Phagocyte abnormalities in some individuals*

- *May have hyperresponsive macrophage/PMNL phenotype, including increased PGE$_2$, IL-1β.*

89

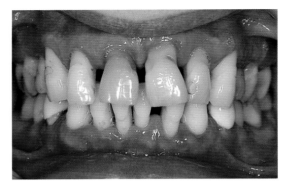

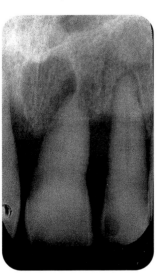

Fig 5-14 Clinical view of generalised aggressive periodontitis in a 27-year-old male (non-smoker). Note the severe generalised inflammation, attachment loss, recession and suppuration around the maxillary incisors.

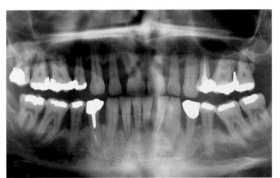

Fig 5-15 Radiographs of the patient in Fig 5-14 showing severe generalised bone loss.

Poorly controlled diabetes

Poorly controlled diabetes can be associated with a more severe form of chronic periodontitis, or, as in this case, aggressive periodontitis, for reasons outlined in Chapters 1 and 3 (Fig 5-16 and Fig 5-17).

Necrotising Periodontal Diseases

Necrotising ulcerative gingivitis (NUG) and necrotising ulcerative periodontitis (NUP) are collectively referred to as necrotising periodontal diseases since they may be different stages of the same infection and there are insufficient

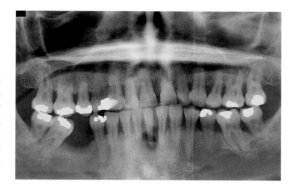

Fig 5-16 Scanora® dentition mode radiograph of patient in her early thirties with poorly controlled type I diabetes and a generalised form of aggressive periodontitis. Note severe bone loss around the mandibular incisor.

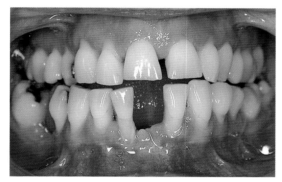

Fig 5-17 The mandibular incisor exfoliated by the time of the next clinical examination.

data to place them in separate categories. NUG can present in young individuals (Fig 5-18). NUG is the only form of bacterial gingivitis presenting with pain. Therefore, the three critical diagnostic features of NUG are:

* pain
* necrosis of the interdental papilla
* bleeding (Box 5-5).

Furthermore, its specific fusiform-spirochaetal bacterial aetiology (*Fusobacteria* spp. and *Treponema* spp: also *Selenomonas* spp and *P. intermedia*) makes it the only type of gingivitis amenable to management with systemic antibiotics (see Chapter 8).

NUG is less common in developed Western societies these days. Stress and malnutrition appear to be contributing more to its occurrence and it is still prevalent in developing countries. There are a number of predisposing factors to the development of NUG:

91

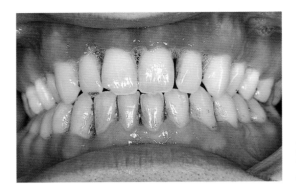

Fig 5-18 Necrotising ulcerative gingivitis in a young male smoker.

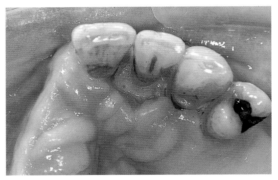

Fig 5-19 Young adult male with AIDS presenting with necrotising ulcerative periodontitis.

- immunosuppression
- stress
- smoking
- malnutrition
- pre-existing gingivitis and poor oral hygiene
- tissue trauma.

NUP manifests as an extension of the necrosis in NUG. It is most commonly seen in individuals with HIV infection (Fig 5-19), severe malnutrition and immunosuppression (Box 5-5).

Box 5-5

Diagnostic Features of Necrotising Periodontal Diseases

Necrotising ulcerative gingivitis (NUG)

- *Three specific features must be present for diagnosis to be made:*
  - *— necrotic ulcers affecting interdental papillae — "punched out"*
  - *— painful ulcers, may be covered by grey slough*
  - *— gingival bleeding with little provocation*
- *Halitosis may be present — characteristic "foetor oris"*
- *Lymph nodes may be involved*
- *Recurrence possible*
- *May progress to NUP*

Necrotising ulcerative periodontitis (NUP)

- *Extension of necrosis to involve periodontal ligament and alveolar bone*

Further considerations

- *May be associated with HIV, immunosuppression (leukaemia), malnutrition*

Abscesses of the Periodontium

There are three types of abscess that can affect the periodontium in younger subjects: the gingival abscess, periodontal abscess and the pericoronal abscess.

Gingival Abscess

A gingival abscess is a localised purulent infection that involves the marginal or interdental papilla (Fig 5-20). Key diagnostic features are shown in Box 5-6.

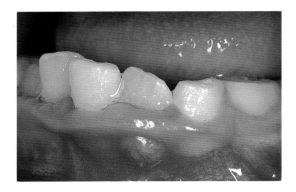

Fig 5-20 Gingival abscess on erupting LL2 in child.

Box 5-6

Diagnostic Features of Gingival Abscess

- *Localised, painful, rapidly expanding swelling*
- *Acute inflammatory response to foreign agents*
- *Red, shiny, smooth swelling*
- *Fluctuant within 24–48 hours*
- *Points and discharges spontaneously*

Periodontal Abscess

The periodontal abscess is the most common type of abscess to affect the periodontium, although not often seen in children. It is defined as a localised purulent infection within the tissues adjacent to the periodontal pocket that may lead to destruction of the periodontal ligament and alveolar bone (Fig 5-21). The descriptor "lateral" was dropped from the terminology of a periodontal abscess following the 1999 International Workshop on Classification as it was felt to be misleading. Common aetiological factors that may aid diagnosis can be elicited from the history:

- Occlusion of the pocket by:
  - impaction of food, foreign body
  - incomplete removal of calculus after recent root surface instrumentation (RSI)
  - bacterial invasion of tissues following recent RSI.
- Furcation involvement.

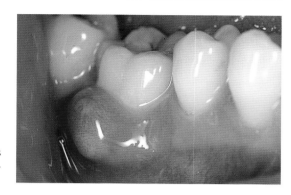

Fig 5-21 Periodontal abscess (LR6) about to point and discharge.

- Poorly controlled diabetes.
- Superinfection with opportunistic organisms following systemic antibiotics.

A thorough examination is needed to support the history and reach a diagnosis. The diagnostic features of a periodontal abscess depend on the stage of formation of the abscess as shown in Box 5-7.

If an acute periodontal abscess is left untreated, it may become chronic – in this case, the pus may discharge through a sinus into the outer gingival surface or via the pocket. Systemic involvement may occur, and this may be another specific indication for systemic antibiotic therapy (Chapter 8).

The differential diagnosis for a periodontal abscess includes:
- Gingival abscess (see Box 5-6).
- Pericoronal abscess (see Box 5-8).
- Periapical abscess (not an abscess of the periodontium).
- Perio-endo lesion (see Box 5-9).

Pericoronal Abscess
This is a localised purulent infection within the tissue surrounding the crown of a partially erupted tooth. It is particularly common around erupting third molars during the late teens and young adulthood (Box 5-8).

Periapical Abscess (not an abscess of the periodontium)
The periapical abscess is not classed as an abscess of the periodontium, but is important in the differential diagnosis of an abscess involving the periodontal tissues. It arises from necrotic pulp tissue, causing an inflammatory

Box 5-7

Diagnostic Features of Periodontal Abscess

Early periodontal abscess formation, pus not draining yet:

- *Pain (may be severe, throbbing)*

- *Vital pulp response*

- *Clinical and radiographic evidence of periodontal involvement:*

  - *pockets*

  - *attachment loss*

  - *bone loss*

  - *furcation may be involved in molars.*

Periodontal abscess with pus to drain:

- *Ovoid elevation of gingiva on lateral aspect of root*

- *Gingiva red and swollen with smooth, shiny surface; feeling of "pressure in gums"; discomfort eases when swelling points and abscess discharges*

- *Suppuration from pocket (gentle pressure)*

- *Mobile tooth*

- *Tooth slightly extruded from socket*

- *Sensation of "wanting to grind tooth"*

- *Vital pulp response*

- *Clinical/radiographic evidence of periodontal involvement (see above).*

Periodontal abscess with systemic involvement — additional features that may present:

- *Extraoral swelling*

- *Lymphadenopathy*

- *Malaise, elevated temperature*

- *Cellulitis (rarely).*

Box 5-8

Diagnostic Features of Pericoronal Abscess

* *Partially erupted tooth*

* *Mandibular third molar common site*

* *Red and swollen gingival flap*

* *Infection may spread*

* *Possible systemic involvement*

---

response in the periapical tissues; the tooth may be heavily restored or have carious pulpal involvement. Therefore, a non-vital pulpal response is a key diagnostic feature of a periapical abscess, and the tooth may be acutely painful and tender to percussion whereas periodontal involvement would not be a feature.

Periodontitis Associated With Endodontic Lesions

There is considerable evidence that communication between the pulp chamber and periodontal ligament occurs through lateral and accessory canals, especially in the bifurcation and trifurcation areas of molars. When the pulp is necrotic, the resulting infection can track through the periodontal tissues, presenting as a narrow periodontal pocket. Conversely, the effect of periodontal inflammation can be detrimental to the pulp via the same lateral canals or the apical foramen. The 1999 International Workshop proposed a category known as the combined periodontal-endodontic lesion (Box 5-9), thereby recognising the interaction of the endodontic and periodontal pathologies, irrespective of the primary source of infection (Fig 5-22a,b). This was first proposed by Chapple and Lumley (1999).

Box 5-9

Periodontitis Associated with Endodontic Lesions (Perio-endo Lesions)

Periodontal features:

- *Increased probing depths adjacent to root surface*
- *Swelling*
- *Bleeding on probing*
- *Increased mobility*
- *Suppuration*
- *Sinus formation*

Endodontic features:

- *Non-vital pulp response*
- *Painful*
- *Tender on percussion*
- *Angular bone loss; may extend around apex; may occur around furcation*
- *May relate to perforations during endodontic root canal therapy*
- *May relate to vertical root fractures*

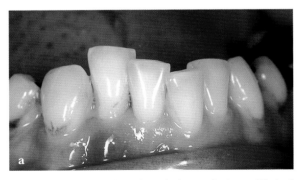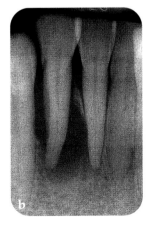

Fig 5-22 (a) Periodontal-endodontic lesion. Clinical view of LR2 showing swelling labially; (b) Radiographic view.

In youngsters, this type of lesion is most likely to occur in response to trauma to incisors, or localised aggressive periodontitis; in the young adult it will most likely be due to aggressive forms of periodontitis or severe cases of chronic periodontitis, particularly where there are confounding risk factors such as tobacco smoking or poorly controlled diabetes. Management is covered in Chapter 8.

Developmental or Acquired Deformities and Conditions

Localised Gingival Recession

Localised gingival recession (LGR) can be the source of much patient concern especially in teenagers and young adults due to the aesthetics and fears of tooth loss (Fig 5-23). Typically, LGR presents on the labial aspect of the lower incisors where the gingival margin may be several millimetres apical to the CEJ, in association with thin gingiva and an underlying bony dehiscence (see Fig 1-10 and Chapple and Gilbert 2002).

Frequently, plaque-induced gingivitis is also present due to the accumulation of plaque around the gingival margin that is located apical to the usual lines of tooth brushing. Concomitant periodontitis can develop secondary to plaque accumulation at such sites, compounding the problems. In addition, a high fraenal attachment can hinder cleaning in the lower incisor region. The BPE will flag the presence of the bleeding (BPE = 1), while supra- and subgingival calculus may also be present (BPE = 2). Recession should be monitored from the gingival margin to the CEJ using a graduated periodontal probe (see Chapter 8); in selected cases it may be necessary to perform a periodontal plastic surgery procedure to prevent progression.

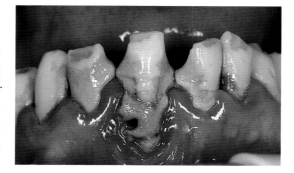

Fig 5-23 A 17-year old female patient with amelogenesis imperfecta and inadequate plaque control around area of localised gingival recession, showing secondary inflammation. Gross deposits of plaque and supragingival calculus are evident.

Occlusal Trauma

Occlusal trauma is injury resulting in tissue changes within the attachment apparatus as a result of occlusal forces. It may be primary (occurring on a tooth without periodontal disease) or secondary (occurring on a tooth with active periodontal disease). The effects of occlusal trauma are more likely to be seen in adulthood than childhood, except where orthodontic problems exist. Occlusal trauma does not initiate gingivitis or periodontitis. Clinical diagnostic features include:

- progressive mobility
- fremitus
- wear facets
- tooth migration
- fractured teeth
- sensitivity.

Radiographically, widened periodontal ligament space, bone loss (furcation, vertical, circumferential) or root resorption may occur.

Key Points

- Plaque-induced forms of gingivitis can affect children, adolescents and young adults.
- It is important to differentiate between chronic periodontitis presenting in adolescents and young adults and aggressive forms of periodontitis.
- The impact of systemic risk factors, such as smoking, stress and poorly controlled diabetes, on all forms of periodontitis needs to be recognised.
- Other periodontal conditions can manifest in the younger age groups and key diagnostic features need to be borne in mind.

References

Chapple ILC, Gilbert AD. Understanding Periodontal Diseases: Assessment and Diagnostic Procedures in Practice. London: Quintessence, 2002:1–16.

Chapple ILC, Lumley PJ. The periodontal-endodontic interface. Dent Update 1999;26:331–341.

Chapter 6

Non-plaque-induced Periodontal Diseases I: Gingival Lesions

Aim

This chapter aims to provide an overview of less common conditions that may present as gingival lesions and which do not have plaque as the primary aetiological agent. Some are gingival manifestations of systemic diseases and some are lesions that are confined to the gingival tissues.

Outcome

Having read this chapter, the practitioner should be able to identify more common non-plaque-induced gingival conditions in young patients, feel empowered to reassure parents and young adults and to manage some of these conditions in their practice. They will also be able to identify key conditions that require specialist referral for further investigation and joint medical/surgical management.

Introduction

The 1999 International Workshop for Classification of Periodontal Diseases used the term "non-plaque-induced" to describe conditions where plaque control measures alone cannot be used to treat a condition (see Chapple and Gilbert 2002 for a critique of the classification). Some of these lesions are relatively common (e.g. childhood viruses), whilst others are extremely rare (see Table 1-1). Many of the conditions do not usually present in younger patients, e.g. those of specific bacterial origin. In contrast, some other non-plaque-induced gingival conditions that may present in the younger age groups were omitted, e.g. granulomatous disease. Therefore a more comprehensive list of the non-plaque-induced gingival conditions that may present in young patients is shown in Table 6-1. The salient features of the more common conditions are briefly discussed below.

Table 6-1 **Non-plaque-induced gingival conditions and lesions in young patients**

Type of lesion	Aetiology	Condition/lesion	GDP/ refer
Infective	*viral*	herpangina	GDP - r
		hand foot and mouth	GDP - r
		herpes simplex I (primary)	GDP - r
		herpes simplex I (secondary)	GDP - r
		molluscum contagiosum	refer
	fungal	candidosis	GDP - r
		linear gingival erythema (candidosis)	refer
	deep mycoses	aspergillosis	refer
		blastomycosis	refer
		coccidiomycosis	refer
		cryptococcosis	refer
		histoplasmosis	refer
		geotricosis	refer
Genetic	*fibromatosis*	hereditary gingival fibromatosis	GDP - r
	coeliac disease	oral/gingival ulceration	refer
	anatomical variations	delayed gingival retreat	GDP
Systemic diseases that manifest within the gingiva	*haematological disease*		
	– benign conditions	agranulocytosis	refer
		cyclical neutropenia	GDP - r
		familial benign neutropenia	GDP - r
		myelodysplastic syndromes	refer
	– malignant conditions	myeloid leukaemia	refer
		b-cell lymphoma	refer
		Hodgkin's lymphoma	refer
	granulomatous inflammations	Crohn's disease	refer
		sarcoidosis	refer
		Melkersson-Rosenthal syndrome	refer
		Wegener's granulomatosis	refer
		tuberculosis	refer
		disseminated pyogenic granulomas	refer
	immunological conditions	hypersensitivity reactions	GDP - r
		lichen planus	refer
		C1-esterase inhibitor deficiency/ dysfunction (angioedema)	refer

Traumatic	*thermal*	burns	GDP
	chemical	ulceration	GDP
	physical	gingivitis artefacta	refer
	electrical	burns	refer

Drug-induced	*immune complex reactions*	erythema multiforme	refer
		lichenoid drug reactions	GDP - r
	cytotoxic drugs	methotrexate	refer
		hydroxychloroquine	refer
	pigmenting drugs drugs	doxycycline	GDP
		oral contraceptives	GDP
		antimalarials	GDP
	anti-retroviral drugs (anti-HIV drugs)	trigeminal nerve neuropathy	refer

GDP, manage in practice.
GDP - r, manage in practice but refer if concerned or complications arise.

Viral Infections

Herpangina

Herpangina is caused by Coxsackie viruses (usually A4 and A10), which are RNA viruses belonging to the picornavirus family. It usually presents within the first few years of life with a prodrome characteristic of viral infections. The baby or child will be irritable, febrile and will have a general malaise with loss of appetite. Cervical lymph nodes enlarge and vesicles, which typ-

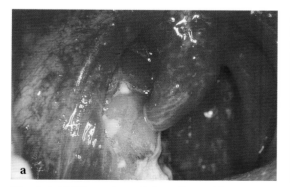
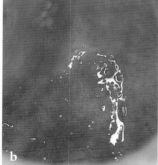

Fig 6-1 (a) Ulceration of the pillars of fauces, soft palate and tonsillar fossa following rupture and coalescence of several vesicles containing coxsackie virus. (b) Vesicles affecting the hard palate adjacent to the upper molar teeth are classic features of herpangina. Vesicles are also present on the soft palate.

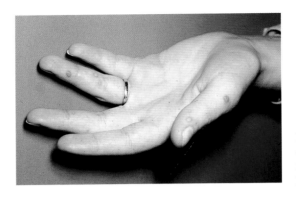

Fig 6-2 Hand, foot and mouth disease often presents with fluid-filled vesicles affecting the palms of the hands.

ify viral infections, appear on the soft palate and fauces (Fig 6-1a,b). These can coalesce and ulcerate causing pain and problems swallowing, but the gingivae are often spared.

It is essential to reassure worried parents that the condition will "burn out" after seven to 10 days. In the meantime, the infant should be adequately hydrated, 0.2% chlorhexidine gently swabbed over areas of ulceration to prevent secondary infection and the use of an analgesic/anti-pyretic elixir (e.g. sugar free paracetamol paediatric syrup) may relieve symptoms. Eating is facilitated by applying topical lidocaine over painful areas or by giving cool fluids to drink. It may be necessary for nocturnal sedation (promethazine hydrochloride for infants over 12 months). Review within seven days to ensure the lesions are resolving and if concerned about dehydration at any time, refer to a paediatric hospital for parenteral feeding.

Complications of herpangina include acute parotitis, which is rare but may be confused with mumps.

Hand, Foot and Mouth Disease
This is caused by Coxsackie virus A16 or occasionally A4, A5, A9 or A10. Transmission is usually faeco-oral. It is very similar to herpangina but skin vesicles appear on the lateral margins of the toes and fingers (Fig 6-2). Oral lesions again present as vesicles affecting the oral mucosa, particularly the soft palate, fauces and non-keratinised mucosa. Vesicles will ulcerate forming small yellow-centred ulcers with a red periphery.

The management is essentially the same as for herpangina, but all attempts should be made to keep the child's hands out of their mouths – easier said

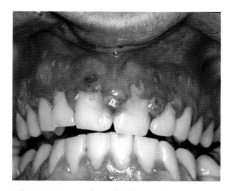

Fig 6-3 Irregular, shallow ulceration of the keratinised gingival margins is a classic sign of herpes simplex infection. The lesions have a ragged margin, yellow base and are very different from those of necrotising ulcerative gingivitis.

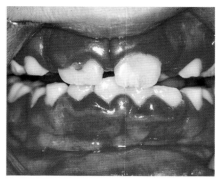

Fig 6-4 Fiery red gingivae with or without ulceration are characteristic of primary herpetic gingivostomatitis. Here, a fibrinous exudate is evident at the gingival margin of the deciduous upper right central incisor.

than done! Complications are also largely the same as for herpangina with dehydration being the main difficulty to guard against.

Herpes Simplex Virus I (HSV-I)

This is a ubiquitous virus and the most common of the eight human herpes viruses. The primary infection may often be subclinical, but symptoms can present with varying severity. The virus remains dormant in the trigeminal ganglion (sacral ganglion in the case of HSV-II which causes genital herpes) and will cause secondary clinical infections when patients feel run down, are immunosuppressed, or following trauma or fever. Recurrent HSV-I affects about 20 – 40% of individuals who have had a primary infection. The most common recurring problem is damage to the lips from ultraviolet light resulting in a "cold sore" (herpes labialis).

Primary Herpetic Gingivostomatitis

HSV-I is the aetiological agent of primary herpetic gingivostomatitis (PHG). PHG usually presents within the first three years of life, but the natural history is changing and reports of onset in teenagers and young adults, in particular, males are becoming more common (Fig 6-3). It is characterised by a prodrome, followed by small vesicles forming throughout the mouth on the oral mucosa, tongue and gingivae. The ulcers coalesce, develop a fibrinous coating and result in a painful stomatitis. The gingivae can appear fiery

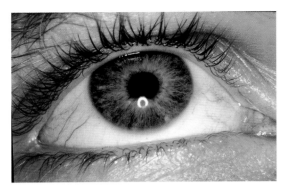

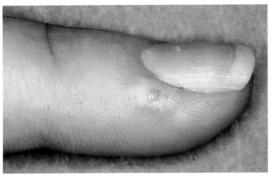

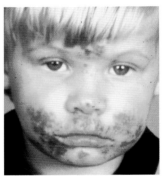

Fig 6-5 A small area of ulceration around the medial canthus of the eye due to HSV-1 transmitted from an oral infection.

Fig 6-6 A herpetic whitlow affecting the forefinger following cross-infection with HSV-1. Such lesions can have serious consequences if osteomyelitis develops as a secondary complication.

Fig 6-7 Herpetic eczema in a young boy following spread from an oral infection. Rarely, a herpetic meningoencephalitis may develop.

red in colour (Fig 6-4), but there are no skin lesions. There may be increased salivation because of pain on swallowing, submandibular lymphadenopathy and a raised temperature.

Management involves supportive therapy as for herpangina, ensuring against dehydration. Review is essential after seven days to ensure that the lesions are resolving and no complications are evident. Complications such as ocular and digit transmission (Figs 6-5 and 6-6) must be guarded against. Rarely, herpetic eczema may develop (Fig 6-7) or in extreme cases a herpetic meningoencephalitis.

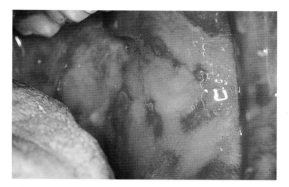

Fig 6-8 Mucosal herpes affecting the buccal mucosa. Ulcers are shallow and irregular with a yellow base, erythema and ragged margins.

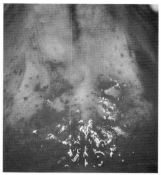

Fig 6-9 Mucosal herpes affecting the hard palate in the same patient as in Fig 6-8.

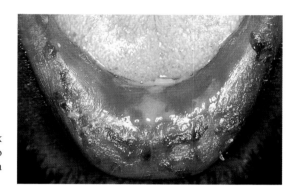

Fig 6-10 Herpes simplex affecting the lips, leading to bleeding and crusting with a fibrinopurulent exudate.

Secondary HSV-I Infection

Herpes labialis

Secondary HSV-I most commonly presents as herpes labialis and can be managed using topical aciclovir cream if diagnosed early. The ideal time to apply topical creams is when the first signs of a cold sore are evident (often a tingling sensation in the lips). Care should be taken treating patients with weeping cold sores, as these contain active virus and can spread with trauma to the lips associated with dental interventions; re-appointment is advisable.

Mucosal or oral herpes

This is the other form of secondary HSV infection. It presents as a viral pro-

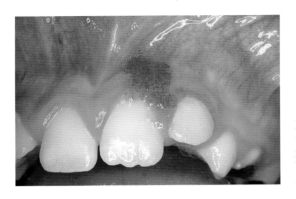

Fig 6-11 A localised lesion of the gingivae around the UL1 in a nine-year-old girl, caused by the pox virus (molluscum contagiosum).

drome of two to four days duration, with flu-like symptoms that may precede the appearance of herpetic ulcers. The prodrome is an important feature when considering differential diagnoses. Oral lesions start as blisters but may go unnoticed until rupture and coalescence into larger erosions affecting the entire oral mucosa, including the hard palate. (Figs 6-8 and 6-9). The gingivae can be sore, swollen and inflamed and the lips may have a bloody, crusted fibrinopurulent exudate (Fig 6-10).

Differential diagnosis of mucosal herpes includes erythema multiforme (see later), herpetiform aphthae, coxsackie virus infections (see earlier) and may rarely indicate leukaemia. A definitive diagnosis can be made from cytology (taking a smear) or more modern methods such as fluorescent antibodies and polymerase chain reaction.

Management largely involves prevention of local and peripheral spread (eyes, fingers – herpetic whitlow) and supportive therapy (bed rest, fluids, topical analgesia). Secondary infection can be prevented with topical application of 0.2% chlorhexidine. If diagnosed early or if severe aciclovir (200mg 5 times daily for five days for children over two years of age and adults; under two years of age give half the adult dose) or valaciclovir (250mg twice daily, **not** recommended for children) taken systemically may help.

Molluscum Contagiosum

This is a rare form of viral wart, which most commonly presents on the skin as a series of raised papules. The virus is a pox virus (distantly related to the small pox virus) and can cause gingival lesions in children who contract the virus at school (Fig 6-11). Always check for skin lesions. Local lesions can be managed by curettage or cryosurgery to prevent distortion of the gingi-

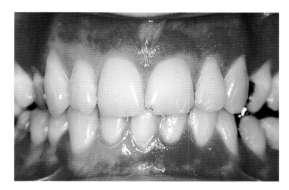

Fig 6-12 Broad band gingival erythema, consistent with a gingival fungal infection with *Candida albicans*.

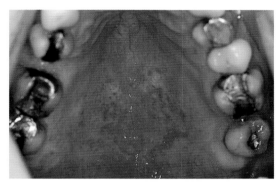

Fig 6-13 Palatal erythematous candidosis caused by a steroid inhaler-induced localised mucosal immunosuppression.

val margin. In young adults lesions may indicate immunosuppression (e.g. HIV infection).

Fungal Infections

Oral fungal infections in younger patients are rare and tend not to manifest gingivally in otherwise healthy patients (Fig 6-12). The most common is candidosis presenting as one of three forms:
• Pseudomembranous candidosis (thrush).
• Erythematous candidosis.
• Chronic hyperplastic candidosis (CHC or plaque-like).

Prevalence of *Candida albicans* is estimated to be as high as 50% in some populations, but several other species (e.g. *C. krusei, C. glabrata, C. dublinienesis*) can also inhabit the oral cavity. The key question to ask with oral candidosis is "Why is it causing infection?". The most common reasons are:

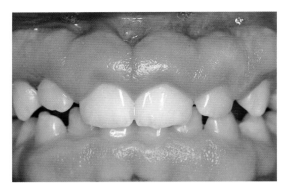

Fig 6-14 Hereditary gingival fibromatosis of the labial gingivae in a 12-year-old boy whose mother, aunt and younger brother were also affected.

- recent course of systemic antibiotics
- intraoral acrylic appliance (partial denture or orthodontic appliance)
- steroid inhalers for asthma. If associated with these it affects the hard palate (Fig 6-13) – give advice to rinse the palate with water after use.
- immunosuppression – undiagnosed or poorly controlled diabetes, or HIV-infection presenting as linear gingival erythema (LGE) or leukaemia are possibilities
- iron deficiency anaemia.

Although the fungal conditions (deep mycoses) listed below can affect the oral mucosa of young patients, they are very rare:
- aspergillosis
- blastomycosis
- coccidiomycosis
- cryptococcosis
- geotricosis
- histoplasmosis (aetiological agent *Histoplasma capsulatum*. It is usually subclinical in healthy patients, the organism being contracted from bird faeces as *H. capsulatum* is a soil saprophyte).

Genetic Conditions

Hereditary Gingival Fibromatosis
Hereditary gingival fibromatosis (HGF) is a rare inherited condition with an autosomal-dominant trait. It usually affects maxillary tuberosities and mandibular retromolar pads; however, labial gingivae can be involved (Fig 6-14). In severe cases eruption and tooth position may be affected and false pocketing may increase the risk of attachment loss. Histologically, a thick-

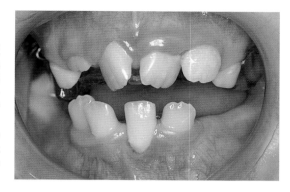

Fig 6-15 Delayed gingival retreat. The gingival margins around all upper incisors and three of the four lower incisors have not reached their mature "adult" position. However, the margin at the LL1 is prematurely at its adult position and may progress to recession.

ened epithelium with prominent rete ridges and dense, thick bundles of collagen fibres are characteristically seen. Management includes gingivectomy for aesthetic and sometimes functional reasons, but extreme care is needed in patients under 16–18 years of age as gingival maturation is not complete (see delayed gingival retreat). Careful plaque control is necessary to prevent recurrence.

Coeliac Disease
This is a gastrointestinal condition arising due to a gluten allergy (wheat protein) and presenting as recurrent oral ulceration. Serologically, it is characterised by increased serum levels of IgG to gliadin, anti-endomysial antibody levels and anti-tissue transglutaminase levels.

Delayed Gingival Retreat
This is a condition in which the erupted tooth has a gingival margin that is coronal to its definitive position above the CEJ (Fig 6-15). Gingivectomy at this stage could be disastrous aesthetically if the gingival margin is still "in retreat".

Systemic Diseases With Gingival Manifestations

Haematological Conditions
Agranulocytosis
This term refers to an extreme neutropenia, which may arise *de novo* or may be drug induced (e.g. by the antithyroid drug carbimazole). Oral signs and symptoms essentially involve recurrent oral ulceration, but the periodontal tissues may also be involved with cyclical or familial benign neutropenia.

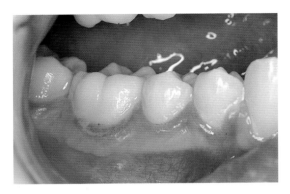

Fig 6-16 Familial benign neutropenia presenting as recurrent gingival ulceration in a 13-year-old girl. Painful marginal ulcerations were similar to, but not caused by, toothbrush trauma.

Cyclical neutropenia
This is a rare condition with cycles of neutrophil depression varying between three and six weeks with an onset early in childhood. Severe gingival inflammation and rapid periodontal breakdown can result, especially around lower incisors and first molars.

Familial benign neutropenia
This rare autosomal dominant condition may present as an ulcerative gingivitis (Fig 6-16) associated with gingival oedema or desquamation. Ulceration of the free gingivae is rare and NUG must be excluded. If mild, management involves symptomatic relief, meticulous oral hygiene and regular prophylaxis. Topical prednesol (prednisolone tablets 10mg twice daily, dissolved in a tumbler of water and used as a mouth rinse) may help, but the condition is often self-limiting within 12–18 months.

Myelodysplastic syndromes
The myelodysplastic syndromes (MDS) are rare haematological disorders of the myeloid cell lineages. They have an incidence of 4:100,000, are heterogeneous in nature and thought to be part of the same spectrum of disorders that give rise to acute myeloid leukaemia (AML). Previously called "pre-leukaemia", MDS have been diagnosed following persistent herpes labialis, severe oral mucosal ulceration and unexplained or spontaneous gingival bleeding inconsistent with plaque levels (Chapple, Saxby, Murray 1999). The incidence of MDS appears to be increasing, and due to the high mortality rates associated with this group of disorders, it is important that the general dental practitioner, who may be the first person to whom patients with MDS present, is aware of its oral manifestations. However, it is highly unlikely that MDS will present in young adults or children, since the age of presentation is usually over 60 years.

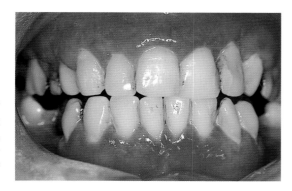

Fig 6-17 A broad "band-like" gingival erythema, with a soft "velvet-like" consistency. Biopsy and subsequent investigation confirmed this to be gingival sarcoidosis.

Leukaemia

Acute forms of leukaemia may present in the under twenties with generalised gingival swelling, following tissue infiltration with the malignant clone of leucocytes (up to 40% of cases), or with spontaneous or excessive bleeding. The bleeding is thought to be due to the thrombocytopenia associated with acute and chronic forms of leukaemia. Investigations involve full blood counts, blood films and gingival biopsy, with acute lymphoblastic leukaemia being the more common form in children.

Granulomatous Inflammations

This diverse group of conditions is characterised by the presence of non-caseating granulomas within the oral mucosa and gingivae. The gingival enlargement can be diffuse, erythematous and granular and feels "velvet-like" to touch (Fig 6-17). They are often collectively, but inaccurately, called the orofacial granulomatoses (OFGs). They are beyond the scope of this chapter and therefore discussion will be brief. They may be due to the following systemic conditions:

- Crohn's disease is of uncertain aetiology and presents as mucosal tags, linear ulceration, a cobblestone appearance of the buccal mucosa and lip swelling with a linear midline fissure (Fig 6-18). There may be a broad band gingival swelling and diagnosis is by biopsy and gastrointestinal investigation of the terminal ileum by sigmoidoscopy and barium imaging methods.
- Sarcoidosis is another of the granulomatous disorders. It is rare (0.02%), more common in Blacks than Caucasians and involves multiple organs and systems (lungs, spleen, liver, eyes, parotid glands and lymph nodes). The gingival manifestations are indistinguishable from other OFGs (see Fig 6-17) and biopsy is needed for identification of granulomas within

113

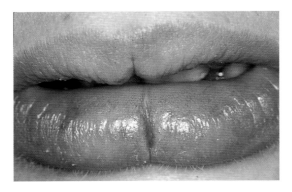

Fig 6-18 Crohn's disease presenting with lip swelling and a midline fissure of the lower lip.

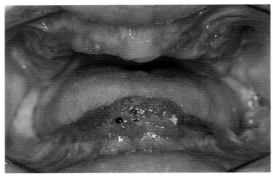

Fig 6-19 Wegener's granulomatosis in an adult, presenting as a strawberry-like granular swelling of the lower alveolus.

the tissues for diagnosis. A chest radiograph may show lung involvement and the granulomas produce angiotensin converting enzyme (ACE), which can be raised in serum. Treatment with steroids has a high success rate.

• Melkersson-Rosenthal syndrome presents in a similar manner to the conditions previously discussed, but classical features are facial oedema/swelling, fissured tongue and a facial nerve palsy.

Wegener's granulomatosis
This is not an OFG, but is nevertheless a systemic disease characterised by a necrotising, granulomatous vasculitis of the respiratory tract (lungs, nose and paranasal sinuses) and kidneys. Lesions can involve the tongue and gingivae, where changes involve a granular "strawberry-like" hyperplasia and ulceration (Fig 6-19). Diagnosis is made following biopsy.

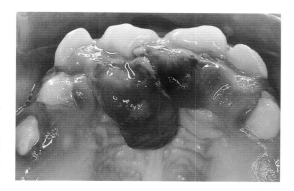

Fig 6-20 An exophytic, vascular enlargement in a seven-year-old boy. Similar lesions were present in the mandible as part of several "disseminated" pyogenic granulomas.

Tuberculosis
The prevalence of tuberculosis has increased in recent years with the HIV epidemic. Multiple drug-resistant forms now exist that are creating serious medical management problems. It is sufficient to say that it is more common in immigrant children who may not have been immunised and thus it should form part of a differential diagnosis when caseating granulomas are evident on biopsy.

Disseminated pyogenic granuloma
This is a rare form of disseminated lobular capillary haemangioma (a pyogenic granuloma). The aetiology is obscure, and it is misnamed, as it is neither infectious nor granulomatous in origin. The granulomas are thought to arise following chronic irritation, or trauma, which stimulates capillary proliferation, sometimes at a rapid rate (within three months). The lesions may appear exophytic, bleed when touched and can necrose like a vascular tumour, however, they are well circumscribed and invasion is not seen. Histologically, they appear identical to a vascular epulis, or localised pyogenic granuloma. The lesion shown in Fig 6-20 was successfully managed by excision, scaling and careful attention to oral hygiene to prevent recurrence.

Immunological Conditions
Hypersensitivity reactions
Hypersensitivity reactions to dietary allergens (e.g. benzoates, cinnamon) give rise to labial and facial swelling, and may cause an angular chelitis and broad band-like gingival inflammation and swelling. Management involves sequential exclusion of putative allergens from the diet.

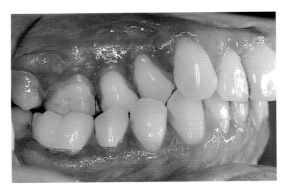

Fig 6-21 Desquamative gingivitis due to lichen planus. Although it has been reported in this age group, lichen planus is extremely rare in children and adolescents.

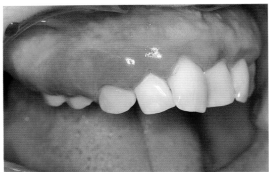

Fig 6-22 Severe gingival oedema in a patient who has C1-esterase inhibitor deficiency (hereditary angioedema – type II). The condition first presented at the age of 17 and is associated with stress.

Lichen planus
Lichen planus is an autoimmune disease of unknown aetiology. It usually presents in the over forties but has been reported in children. It can present as a desquamative gingivitis (Fig 6-21) where eroded patches appear beneath areas of white desquamating epithelium. This will be discussed in more detail in the fifth book of this series (Chapple and Hamburger), but young adults presenting with this condition should be referred to exclude drug-induced lichenoid reactions or underlying systemic (e.g. liver) disease.

C1-esterase inhibitor deficiency/dysfunction
The clinical term for this condition is angioedema, which may be hereditary (HAO) or acquired in nature. It involves a defect in an enzyme that damps down complement activation (see Chapple and Gilbert 2002). The acquired form usually presents in adults but HAO, which has an autosomal dominant pattern of inheritance, can present in younger patients. Classically, it presents with lip swelling, or angioedema of the head, neck or extremi-

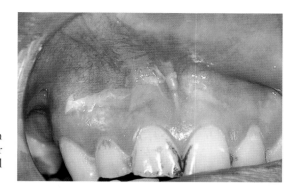

Fig 6-23 A chemical burn affecting the reflected sulcular mucosa caused by the local application of aspirin.

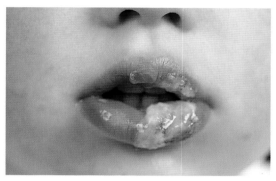

Fig 6-24 An electrical burn of the lips in a two-year-old child who bit into an electrical cable in her father's garage.

ties. Additionally, oedema of the tongue, cheeks and upper airway often leads to breathlessness, which can, in severe cases, be life threatening. HAO is classified into type I (a decrease in production of enzyme) or type II (normal levels but dysfunctional enzyme). Chapple and colleagues have recently reported type II HAO localised to the gingivae (Fig 6-22), which presented initially at the age of 17 years in a young female. However, medical and surgical management is complex and referral is recommended.

Traumatic Lesions

These include lesions such as:
- Chemical ulceration – arising most commonly from the local use of aspirin or toothache tinctures adjacent to an area of dental pain (Fig 6-23).
- Thermal burns – more commonly affect the palate or tongue.
- Electrical burns – extremely rare but may arise in very young children (Fig 6-24).

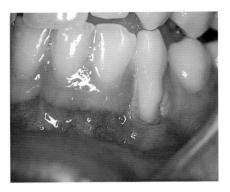

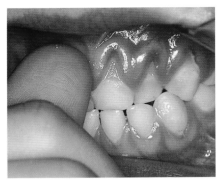

Fig 6-25a Factitious injury – known as gingivitis artefacta, caused by finger nail picking of the gingival margins by an adolescent female who was seeking attention. The attachment loss around the LL3 is significant and marginal keratinisation of the gingivae is consistent with chronic trauma.

Fig 6-25b Gingivitis artefacta in a teenager demonstrating how the trauma is caused.

- Physical trauma – there are many forms of physical trauma ranging from accidental and habitual injury, to factitious injury in cases such as gingivitis artefacta (Fig 6-25a,b). The latter condition is more common amongst teenage females and is a manifestation of attention seeking behaviour. The fingernail is often used to scratch the gingival tissues, which recede and attachment loss can reach extreme proportions where teeth can exfoliate. A related condition is obsessive-compulsive disorder where patients can become obsessed with the gingival tissues and deliberately try to disfigure them (Fig 6-26). Care is needed when arranging management for such children and young adults, as there may often be a need for counselling or even psychiatric referral.

Drug-induced Lesions

Erythema Multiforme

Erythema multiforme is a rare condition believed to be a form of hypersensitivity reaction to antigens (e.g. previous HSV-I infection) or mitogens (certain drugs can cause it, e.g. antimicrobials), and which results in vesiculobullous eruptions affecting the oral mucosa. They have an erythematous

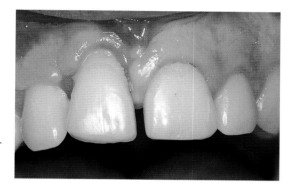

Fig 6-26 A 17-year-old male clinically diagnosed with obsessive-compulsive disorder attacked his gingival margin above UR1 with a pair of scissors leading to marked recession.

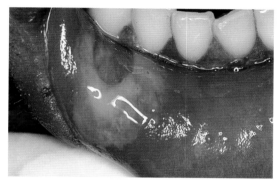

Fig 6-27 Labial erythema multiforme in a 15-year-old male who also had genital lesions as part of the Stevens-Johnson syndrome. The reaction was believed to be due to medication with prednisolone, which when withdrawn led to resolution of the lesions.

margin and shallow mucosal erosions may also arise (Fig 6-27). The lips can have a crusted fibrinopurulent surface and there may be ocular and genital lesions as well as classical skin lesions called target lesions. Features which distinguish erythema multiforme from HSV I infection are:

- Sparing of the gingiva from ulceration.
- No prodrome.
- There may be no regional lymphadenopathy.
- Genital involvement is unlikely with HSV-I in patients who are not sexually mature.
- Target lesions (iris lesions) on the skin (Fig 6-28).

A severe form of erythema multiforme exists called Stevens-Johnson syndrome and management often involves systemic steroids and local analgesic preparations for relief of symptoms.

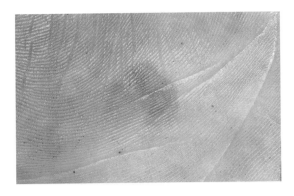

Fig 6-28 A so-called "target lesion" on the skin of the patient in Fig 6-27.

Cytotoxic Drugs

Cytotoxic drugs like methotrexate are being used more commonly as part of the aggressive management of juvenile arthritis and can cause bone marrow suppression and gingival ulceration (Fig 6-29).

Pigmenting Drugs

Pigmenting drugs may give rise to local lesions, including gingival freckles (gingival ephylis), induced by oral contraceptives or to more generalised pigmentation, associated with antimalarials and some antibiotics. The patient in Fig 6-30 presented with "purple" gingivae and mucosal tissues following long-term use of doxycycline for acne.

Anti-retroviral Drugs

Anti-retrovirals used in the management of HIV-disease have many side effects, including:

- oral ulceration [due to bone marrow suppression, e.g. zidovudine (AZT), zalcitabine (ddC)]
- xerostomia [e.g. didanosine (ddl)]
- trigeminal neuropathies
- gingival bleeding (due to thrombocytopenia).

Specialist referral is advised for the management of these conditions.

Key Points

- Non-plaque-induced gingival diseases/lesions are relatively common in children, adolescents and young adults.

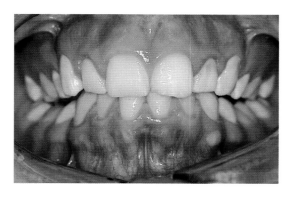

Fig 6-29 Gingival ulceration induced by the cytotoxic drug methotrexate, used in the management of aggressive rheumatoid arthritis in a 16-year-old girl.

Fig 6-30 This 19-year-old girl presented with a complaint of "purple gums", which had resulted from a protracted course of minocycline therapy for teenage acne.

- Non-plaque-induced gingival conditions and lesions in younger patients may represent:
  - an infective origin
  - a genetic origin
  - underlying systemic diseases
  - episodes of trauma
  - adverse reactions to a variety of drugs.
- Childhood viruses may frequently affect the gingival tissues and require careful monitoring to ensure against dehydration or local/systemic spread. Most, however, resolve spontaneously within two weeks and simply require supportive care and parental counselling and reassurance.
- If underlying genetic or systemic diseases are suspected, early specialist referral is advisable.
- Drug-induced lesions are difficult to diagnose and management should involve close liaison with the medical team. Drug-induced lichenoid reactions are rare in children because they are most commonly caused

by drugs used for managing adult diseases (e.g. β-blockers, non-steroidal anti-inflammatory drugs – NSAIDs).

References

Chapple ILC, Gilbert AD. Understanding Periodontal Diseases: Assessment and Diagnostic Procedures in Practice. London: Quintessence, 2002.

Chapple ILC, Saxby MS, Murray J. Gingival haemorrhage, myelodysplastic syndromes and acute myeloid leukaemia. J Periodontol 1999;70:1247–1253.

Further Reading

Chapple ILC. Periodontal diseases in children and adolescents: classification, aetiology and management. Dent Update 1996;23:210–216.

Meyle J, Gonzales JR. Influences of systemic diseases on periodontitis in children and adolescents. Periodontol 2000 2001;26:92–112.

Roberts A, Shah M, Chapple ILC. C-1 esterase inhibitor dysfunction localised to the periodontal tissues: clues to the role of stress in the pathogenesis of chronic periodontitis? J Clin Periodontol 2003;30:271–277.

Seymour RA, Heasman PH (Eds.) Drugs, Diseases and the Periodontium. Oxford: Oxford Medical Publications, 1992.

Chapter 7

Non-plaque-induced Periodontal Diseases II: Periodontal Lesions

Aim

The aim of this chapter is to raise the awareness of practitioners of the rare systemic diseases that may, as part of their clinical course, give rise to severe periodontal destruction. Fortunately, there are relatively few conditions that may present in this manner.

Outcome

It is anticipated that, having read this chapter, the practitioner will bear in mind the need to examine the primary, mixed and secondary dentitions for signs of periodontal destruction. In addition, the reader will be able to recognise the periodontal hallmarks of underlying systemic diseases and refer for specialist management with an appropriate degree of priority.

Introduction

The 1999 International Workshop Classification for Periodontal Diseases (see Chapple and Gilbert 2002) broadly classifies systemic diseases with periodontal manifestations as those of:
- genetic origin
- haematological origin
- not otherwise specified.

In this chapter, "not otherwise specified" is not discussed but Connective tissue disorders are discussed (Table 7-1).

Genetic Conditions with Periodontal Manifestations

Down Syndrome
Down syndrome is an inherited autosomal disorder that results from trisomy of chromosome 21. Approximately 50–90% of patients suffer from destructive periodontal disease, affecting both primary and secondary dentitions and an increased incidence of necrotising ulcerative gingivitis (NUG) has been reported. The lower incisors and upper molars are most commonly affected,

Table 7-1 **Non plaque-induced conditions and lesions in young patients affecting the periodontal attachment**

Aetiology	Condition	Subcategory	GDP/ refer
Genetic disorders	Down syndrome		GDP-r
	type 1 diabetes		GDP-r
	Papillon-Lefèvre syndrome		refer
	Ehlers–Danlos syndrome	type IV	refer
		type VIII	refer
	hypophosphatasia	perinatal	refer
		infantile	refer
		childhood	refer
		adult	refer
	Cohen syndrome		refer
	Job syndrome		refer
	glycogen storage disease		refer
Haematological disorders			
White blood cell disorders	Infantile genetic agranulocytosis		refer
	Leukocyte adhesion deficiency		refer
	Lazy leukocyte syndrome		refer
	Chédiak-Higashi syndrome		refer
	agamma/hypogamma-globulinaemia		refer
	Chronic granulomatous disease		refer
	Histiocytosis-x	Hand-Schüller-Christian disease	refer
		Letterer-Siwe disease	refer
		eosinophilic granuloma	refer
	lymphocyte deficiencies – t-cell	DiGeorge syndrome	refer
	lymphocyte deficiencies – t- and b-cell	Wiskott-Aldrich syndrome	refer
Red blood cell disorders	acatalasia		refer
	aplastic anaemia		refer
Connective tissue disorders	scleroderma	systemic sclerosis	refer
		morphoea (localised)	refer

GDP-r, manage in practice but refer if concerned or problems arise.
Refer, refer to periodontal specialist for advice and treatment.

and the propensity for shortened roots can result in early tooth loss. The underlying pathobiology is believed to involve neutrophil (polymorphonuclear leucocyte – PMNL) defects of chemotaxis, phagocytosis and killing, depressed T-cell-induced antigen killing and abnormal collagen biosynthesis. Care should be taken when planning periodontal therapy, since cardiac defects requiring antibiotic prophylaxis are very common in patients with Down syndrome.

Type 1 Diabetes

The incidence of Type I diabetes in Europe varies between 0.03% and 0.005%. However, data regarding the incidence of periodontitis in diabetic children and non-diabetic controls are conflicting. There appears to be an increased susceptibility to gingival inflammation in younger type 1 diabetics with poor glucose control in comparison to those with good control or non-diabetic subjects (see Chapter 3). However, the data for an increased risk of periodontitis are not as convincing.

Papillon–Lefèvre Syndrome

Papillon-Lefèvre syndrome (PLS) is an inherited autosomal dominant disorder, more common in consanguineous families. Thus, some Indian and Pakistani children may be affected more than Caucasians. The gene defect was recently mapped to the long arm of chromosome 11 (11q) and results in the loss of function of an important PMNL enzyme called cathepsin-C. Cathepsin-C is a lysosomal enzyme found in the primary granules of PMNLs that is important for bacterial destruction and is expressed in the skin of the feet and hands. PLS affects one to four patients per million and the classic signs are usually apparent by two to four years of age:

- Palmar-plantar keratosis (Fig 7-1 and 7-2).
- Rapidly progressive periodontal breakdown affecting both primary and secondary dentitions and leading to premature tooth loss (Figs 7-3 and 7-4).
- Intracranial calcifications (sometimes reported).

The infant presents with severe gingival inflammation with or without recession and tooth mobility (Fig 7-3). Bone loss is severe and rapidly progressive, often leading to total deciduous tooth loss by four years of age. The inflammation resolves during the edentulous phase, consistent with a microbial aetiology, and returns with the eruption of the permanent dentition. Frequently, complete loss of the adult dentition results by early to mid-teens.

Diagnosis of PLS is largely based on clinical signs and symptoms and a thor-

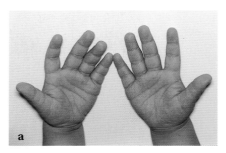
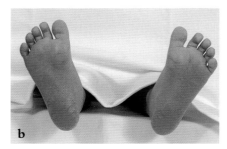

Fig 7-1 Keratosis affecting (a) the palms of the hands and (b) the soles of the feet of a two-year-old boy with Papillon Lefèvre syndrome. The gene mutation was a common mutation (R272P).

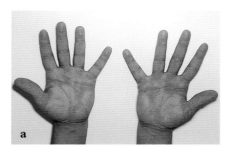
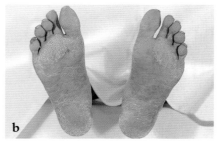

Fig 7-2 Keratosis affecting (a) the palms of the hands and (b) the soles of the feet of the father of the child in Fig 7-1.

ough family history. Genetic diagnosis is now offered in specialist laboratories, and referral is recommended. Symptoms do appear to decrease with age, irrespective of oral hygiene standards, but this is usually too late to save the dentition.

Treatment strategies for PLS vary widely, which is also true for success rates. Most reports have demonstrated poor efficacy of both surgical and non-surgical therapy, though strict plaque control can slow down the progression of the disease. Recent reports have indicated improvement in success rates by:

- Extraction of all deciduous teeth to provide a period of edentulousness.
- Scaling and root surface instrumentation of permanent teeth in conjunction with systemic antibiotics.
- Biweekly professional prophylaxis and repeated mechanical therapy after identification of *A. actinomycetemcomitans*.

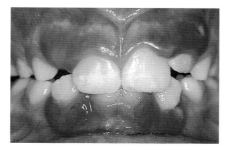

Fig 7-3 Severe gingival inflammation in a seven-year-old boy with Papillon Lefèvre syndrome whose anterior teeth had grade II mobility.

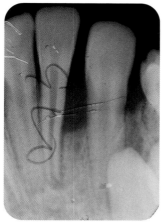

Fig 7-4 Substantial bone loss affecting the permanent incisors of the patient in Fig 7-3.

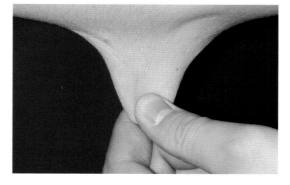

Fig 7-5 Ehlers Danlos syndrome: skin hyperextensibility.

Ehlers–Danlos Syndrome

Ehlers–Danlos syndrome is an autosomal dominant disorder with 10 subcategories, essentially involving defective collagen synthesis. Types IV (autosomal dominant/recessive) and VIII (autosomal dominant) are associated with destructive periodontitis, consistent clinically with a generalised aggressive periodontitis. Systemically there is:
- extensive joint mobility
- skin hyperextensibility (Fig 7-5)
- excessive bruising due to fragile blood vessels.

Clinical signs other than aggressive periodontitis include gingival haemorrhage on brushing and following periodontal therapy or extractions, and poor healing. Referral is essential to facilitate definitive subcategorisation because type IV can be life-threatening.

Hypophosphatasia

Hypophosphatasia is a rare heritable enzymopathy in which a defect exists in one of the major isoforms of the enzyme alkaline phosphatase (ALP). ALP is the enzyme responsible for skeletal and dental mineralisation and the spectrum of disease that results from mutations in the ALP gene has resulted in five clinical subtypes:

- Perinatal (or lethal) – infants live only a few days (rachitic chest leads to respiratory failure).
- Infantile – presents with systemic manifestations in the first six months of life (wide fontanelles, blue sclera, flail chest, poor feeding/weight gain).
- Childhood – see below.
- Adulthood – see below.
- Pseudohypophosphatasia or odontohypophosphatasia – see below.

The condition affects all racial groups with an incidence of 1:100,000 and there is evidence for inheritance in an autosomal dominant form, which produces milder phenotypic features and an autosomal recessive form with severe phenotypic features.

Childhood hypophosphatasia is the most common form seen by dentists. Its features are:

- Premature deciduous tooth loss due to cementum hypoplasia or aplasia.
- Horizontal bone loss, due to disuse atrophy (no cementum link with periodontal ligament; Fig 7-6).
- No root resorption, teeth often exfoliate with complete roots.
- Bone involvement (rickets) can lead to short stature and delayed walking or bone pain.
- Wide open fontanelles may be a feature.
- Proptosis (bulging eyes) due to premature fusion of cranial sutures and increasing intracranial pressure.
- "Beaten copper" appearance to calvarium (often appears like "punched out" lesions).

Adult hypophosphatasia is generally diagnosed during middle age. It is milder in form and may present with a history of early deciduous tooth loss and loss of the six permanent maxillary and mandibular incisor teeth. There may be bone pain and a history of stress fractures (for detailed review see Chapple 1993).

Odontohypophosphatasia has been largely localised to the teeth, with the

128

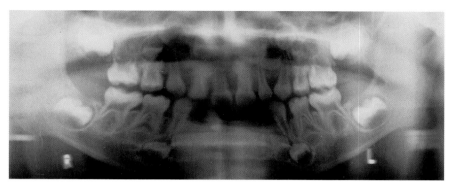

Fig 7-6 Radiographic evidence of premature deciduous tooth loss in a five-year-old boy with hypophosphatasia.

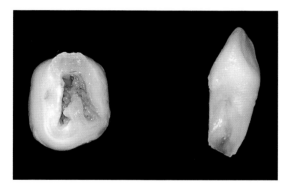

Fig 7-7 Enlarged pulp chambers of teeth that spontaneously exfoliated from the patient in Fig 7-6.

lower deciduous anterior teeth being the most prone to exfoliation, often with intact roots, although root resorption is reported. Other features include enlarged pulp chambers (Fig 7-7).

Diagnosis of hypophosphatasia is complex and involves demonstration of reduced plasma ALP levels and raised levels of certain ALP substrates, e.g. increased phosphoethanolamine in urine and increased pyridoxal-5-phosphate in plasma. Chapple *et al.* (1992) have diagnosed a case with crevicular fluid ALP analysis using a highly sensitive assay developed in their laboratories. Although management is medical in nature, it is vital to maintain excellent oral hygiene and to reduce local risk factors for periodontitis to a minimum.

Cohen Syndrome

Cohen syndrome is inherited in an autosomal recessive manner and is characterised by:

- extensive alveolar bone loss (possibly associated with a neutropenia)
- mental retardation
- motor function defects
- obesity
- dysmorphia.

Job Syndrome

Named after Job of the Old Testament, this is a very rare syndrome that involves hyperimmunoglobulinaemia (IgE) and excessive histamine release by mast cells. Clinically, it presents with severe gingivitis and early onset periodontitis. Children may present with skin rashes, although the main sign is delayed root resorption and loss of deciduous teeth, thus resulting in delayed eruption of the permanent dentition.

Glycogen Storage Disease

The glycogen storage diseases are a series of five conditions characterised by an inability to metabolise or break down glycogen. Type 1B is autosomal recessive and patients are neutropenic with defective neutrophil function and associated periodontal disease.

Haematological Disorders

Haematological disorders with periodontal manifestations in young patients can be divided into those that affect white blood cells and those that affect red blood cells.

Disorders of the White Blood Cells

Infantile genetic agranulocytosis
This is a rare autosomal recessive disorder that involves a severe neutropenia and is characterised by an aggressive periodontitis.

Leukocyte adhesion deficiency
This is a rare autosomal recessive disorder that is characterised by defects in the adhesion molecules that are fundamental for leucocyte recruitment to areas of infection (see Chapple and Gilbert 2002). Severe periodontal disease is described in young patients and the disorder can be life-threatening in the event of septicaemia resulting from a general susceptibility to infection. The defects affect LFA-1 and MAC-1 receptors (see Chapple and

Gilbert 2002) and types I and II have been described. Deciduous teeth exfoliate early and a pre-pubertal periodontitis affects the permanent dentition.

Lazy leucocyte syndrome
This rare condition largely affects the gingiva rather than the periodontal attachment. It is characterised by defective PMNL chemotaxis.

Chédiak-Higashi syndrome
This is a rare autosomal recessive condition, which largely affects PMNL and monocyte function. Defects include:
- impaired chemotaxis
- defective bacterial killing
- defective degranulation
- hyperresponsive phagocytes.

Oral manifestations include:
- severe gingival inflammation
- suppurative periodontitis with tooth mobility
- oral ulceration
- early deciduous tooth loss
- severe periodontal bone loss.

Various treatment regimes have been described, including vitamin C supplementation, cytotoxic drugs (e.g. methotrexate, vincristine) and corticosteroids.

Agamma/hypogammaglobulinaemia
Agamma/hypogammaglobulinaemia is characterised by deficiencies in IgG_2 or IgG_4 and has been reported to be associated with destructive periodontitis.

Chronic granulomatous disease
Chronic granulomatous disease (CGD) is reported to occur in autosomal and x-linked recessive forms. The respiratory burst that creates superoxide and other free radicals fails with the result that bacteria, although phagocytosed by PMNLs rather than being destroyed, are released in a viable state. Unsurprisingly, sufferers have severely compromised infection control mechanisms rendering them susceptible to osteomyelitis and pneumonia. Reported periodontal manifestations seem to be limited to severe gingival inflammation and ulceration, rather than periodontal destruction, which is surprising.

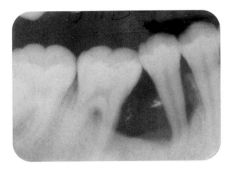

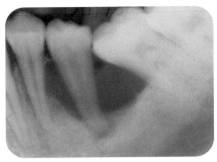

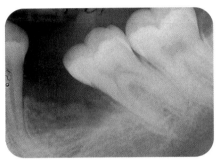

Fig 7-8 Histiocytosis-X presenting as severe localised bone loss around the mandibular second premolars in a 14-year-old boy.

Fig 7-9 Post-extraction healing (same patient as in Fig 7-8) following chemotherapy for the histiocytosis.

Histiocytosis-X
There are three subtypes of histiocytosis-X:
• Hand-Schüller Christian disease
• Letterer-Siwe disease
• eosinophilic granuloma.

The two former subtypes have a malignant course, but eosinophilic granuloma is normally a benign lesion of bone, which can affect the overlying gingivae. All three subtypes more commonly affect the mandible than maxilla, with gingival bleeding, pocketing and severe bone loss reported. Tissue collections of histiocytes and eosinophils characterise the condition histologically. The 14-year-old boy in Fig 7-8 presented with an exophytic gingival swelling adjacent to the second premolars and severe, localised vertical bone loss and tooth mobility. He responded well to local non-surgical periodontal management in conjunction with systemic cytotoxic drug therapy. However, extraction of the premolars became necessary to provide a definitive, stable and manageable result in the long term (Fig 7-9).

Lymphocyte deficiencies – T-cell
DiGeorge syndrome is a rare primary immune deficiency disease, largely affecting T-lymphocyte function, the cause being a gene deletion from the long arm of chromosome 22. Various facial abnormalities have been reported, including cleft palate. An early-onset form of periodontitis has also been described.

Lymphocyte deficiencies – T- and B-cell
Wiskott-Aldrich syndrome is an X-linked immune deficiency involving a deficiency of T and B-cells and thrombocytopenia.

Disorders of the Red Blood Cells
Acatalasia
Acatalasia is a deficiency of the antioxidant enzyme catalase, which is important for preventing damage to red blood cells by hydrogen peroxide produced during metabolism, or as a product of the respiratory burst. The deficiency can lead to oxidation of haemoglobin, decreased oxygen carriage, tissue ischaemia and gingival necrosis. Severe periodontitis has also been reported in adolescents, presumably as a result of excessive oxygen radical damage (in the absence of catalase) leading to connective tissue attachment loss and bone loss.

Aplastic anaemia
Aplastic anaemia is a bone marrow disorder in which fat replaces haematopoietic tissue causing anaemia, neutropenia and thrombocytopenia. Case reports of periodontal manifestations are rare and include gingival bleeding and severe destructive periodontitis.

Disorders of the Connective Tissues

Progressive Systemic Sclerosis
Progressive systemic sclerosis (systemic scleroderma or systemic sclerosis) is a connective tissue disorder of unknown aetiology, which typically affects women of 30 to 60 years of age and is therefore not discussed further.

Localised Scleroderma
Localised or linear scleroderma (morphoea) is predominantly a cutaneous disease. The aetiology has been claimed to have a genetic component or it may arise following trauma. Baxter *et al.* (2001) described the case of a 12-year-old female patient, who initially presented with localised gingival retraction and root exposure affecting UR1 and UR2 (Fig 7-10). The case had

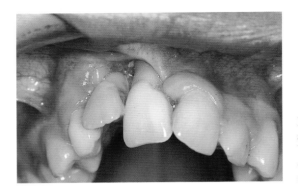

Fig 7-10 Localised recession and scarring around UR1 and UR2, as a result of a condition called morphoea (localised scleroderma).

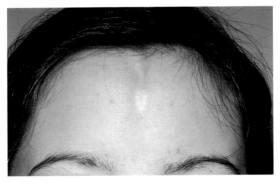

Fig 7-11 A midline *coupe de sabre* in the same patient as in Fig 7-10, which was hidden by a fringe.

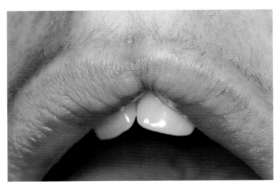

Fig 7-12 Midline notching of the upper lip in the patient from Fig 7-10.

been referred for connective tissue grafting, but careful examination revealed a linear *coupe de sabre* (linear cut of the sword) or linear morphoea, hidden beneath the girl's fringe (Fig 7-11) and midline notching of the upper lip (Fig 7-12). The periodontal condition was managed conservatively for four years, but when the patient was 16 and aesthetics became an important factor in her life, she opted for extraction and prosthetic replacement of UR1 and UR2. A lip split and contour revision was also performed and future fixed prostheses are planned (with or without implant retainers).

General Management Issues Surrounding Non-plaque-induced Periodontal Conditions

The destructive and often complex nature of the non-plaque-induced periodontal conditions and their potential for being a window for underlying systemic diseases should alert the practitioner to make prompt referrals for specialist periodontal advice and treatment (see Chapter 10). It may be difficult to make a definitive diagnosis and instigate appropriate therapy without specialist help for the periodontal lesion that occurs rarely. It is critical to liaise fully with the medical team involved in caring for the young patient (Chapter 9). Once the periodontal problems have been stabilised, the dental practitioner and the dental team can play an important role in periodontal maintenance (Chapter 8).

Key Points

- Non-plaque-induced periodontal conditions and lesions in young individuals can arise from various systemic disorders of genetic, haematological or connective tissue origin.
- Severe periodontal destruction can occur rapidly in some of these young patients.
- Diagnosis of some of the rarer non-plaque-induced periodontal conditions and lesions can be difficult.
- Prompt referral for specialist advice and treatment should be sought where necessary.

References

Baxter AM, Roberts A, Shaw L, Chapple ILC. Localised scleroderma in a 12-year-old girl presenting as gingival recession. A case report and literature review. Dent Update 2001;28:458–462.

Chapple ILC. Hypophosphatasia: dental aspects and mode of inheritance. J Clin Periodontol 1993;20:615–622.

Chapple ILC, Thorpe GHG, Smith JM, et al. Hypophosphatasia: a family study involving a case diagnosed from gingival crevicular fluid. J Clin Periodontol 1992;21:426–431.

Further Reading

Chapple ILC, Gilbert AD. Understanding Periodontal Diseases: Assessment and Diagnostic Procedures in Practice. London: Quintessence, 2002.

Seymour RA, Heasman P.H (Eds.) Drugs, Diseases and the Periodontium. Oxford: Oxford Medical Publications, 1992.

Chapter 8

Principles and Phases of Treatment

Aim

This chapter highlights the principles and phases of periodontal treatment that should be provided for young patients with periodontal diseases.

Outcome

After reading this chapter the practitioner should be aware of how to plan periodontal therapy for the young patient. The reader should have a general understanding of the stages of periodontal treatment (initial, corrective and supportive) and the management of acute periodontal conditions.

Phases of Treatment

When planning periodontal therapy it is useful to consider the management across three phases:
- initial
- corrective
- supportive.

There may be some overlap of procedures and differences in the length of the three phases for different patients and the endpoint of a specific phase of treatment may not always be clear. Nevertheless, such division helps to organise the treatment, to plan what procedures are to be undertaken by which members of the dental team (see Chapter 10) and to avoid missing any key stages of therapy.

Initial Therapy

This is the first phase in the management and is critical to the success of treatment. It is geared to controlling the primary causative factor in periodontal disease, which is plaque. Even in more complex cases where some of the therapy may be provided by a specialist periodontist this phase of treatment can usually be provided in general dental practice, unless there are medical contraindications. The steps that constitute the initial phase of therapy are shown in Fig 8-1.

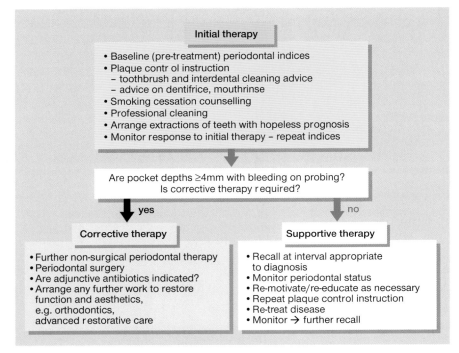

Fig 8-1 Components of initial, corrective and supportive phases of periodontal therapy.

Baseline Measurements

The clinician needs to have a record of the extent of disease and the teeth and sites that are affected against which the progress of treatment can be monitored. The Basic Periodontal Examination (BPE) will indicate sextants or index teeth in the mouth where shallow or deep pockets exist. Use of the code ★ (in addition to the sextant or index tooth score) will flag the presence of furcation defects or clinical attachment loss of 7mm or more. A detailed examination, using appropriate indices (see Chapple and Gilbert 2002), should be done for the following if a BPE score of 4 or ★ is recorded:

- probing pocket depths (PPD) (essential)
- clinical attachment levels (necessary in some cases)
- bleeding on probing (essential)
- mobility (essential)
- furcation involvement (essential)
- suppuration (essential)
- recession (necessary in some cases).

A detailed baseline chart should also be considered for BPE score 3 in young patients in whom identification of early disease is crucial but difficult due to the mixed dentition stage delayed gingival retreat, etc. The probing pocket depth and clinical attachment level measures are described in Box 8-1.

Box 8-1

Probing pocket depths
- *Measured in millimetres with graduated probe*
- *Six sites for each tooth (mesiobuccal, mid-buccal, distobuccal, mesiopalatal, mid-palatal, distopalatal)*
- *Measured from base of pocket to gingival margin*

Clinical attachment levels
- *Measured in millimetres with graduated probe*
- *Six sites for each tooth*
- *Measured from base of pocket to cemento-enamel junction*

Although individual probing pocket depths should be recorded for all young patients with evidence of true pocketing from the BPE score, attachment level measurements may not always be made. Attachment levels can be difficult to measure as the position of the cemento-enamel junction (CEJ) is not always easy to detect. However, because the attachment level is measured from a fixed point it can provide the clinician with valuable information on degree of disease which is not dependent on the variable position of the gingival margin. A number of factors can affect the probing pocket depth and attachment level measurements:
- force applied (ideally 0.20–0.25 N or 20–25g)
- probe diameter (commonly 0.5mm)
- inflammation of tissues (the greater the inflammation, the greater the risk of over probing)
- position of gingival margin (probing pocket depths only)
- presence of calculus (may block probe advancement)
- angulation of probe
- position of probe at gingival margin
- access
- crown form
- patient tolerance
- visual interpretation and reading of probe gradations by the operator (manual probes only).

The measures and indices for bleeding on probing, furcation involvement, suppuration and recession are shown in Box 8-2.

Box 8-2

Bleeding on probing
- *Probing performed to base of pocket*
- *Six sites for each tooth (mesiobuccal, mid-buccal, distobuccal, mesiopalatal, mid-palatal, distopalatal)*
- *Presence of bleeding from base of pocket recorded on chart*

Mobility
- *Light force applied with handles of two instruments – do not use finger pressure*
- *Grade I = up to 1mm movement horizontally*
- *Grade II = more than 1mm movement horizontally*
- *Grade III = movement of tooth both horizontally and vertically*

Furcation involvement (Fig 8-2)
- *Probe around multirooted tooth to detect horizontal bone loss between roots*
- *F 1 = horizontal loss of periodontal support not exceeding one-third of the buccolingual width of the tooth*
- *F 2 = horizontal loss of periodontal support exceeding one-third of the width of the tooth, but not encompassing the total width of the furcation area*
- *F 3 = through and through between two roots*

Suppuration
- *Record sites with presence of suppuration on probing*

Recession
- *Measured in millimetres with graduated probe*
- *Measure from apically placed gingival margin to cemento-enamel junction*
- *Record specific sites where recession noted*

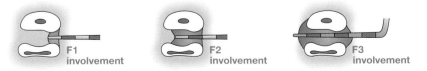

Fig 8-2 Diagram illustrating the degrees of furcation involvement.

Other Baseline Measurements

Plaque and marginal gingival bleeding

The major aetiological agent in periodontal diseases is plaque and therefore treatment has to be directed at its removal and preventing its re-formation. In view of this, two further types of measure are relevant to the management of young patients with BPE scores of 1 and 2 who have gingivitis, as well as for those showing signs of periodontitis. These are plaque and marginal gingival bleeding scores, which are recorded at baseline to evaluate the level of plaque control the patient has been able to achieve without instruction (Box 8-3). The scores are then repeated as required to monitor the patient's oral hygiene and motivation. Marginal gingival bleeding scores provide a better measure of longer-term plaque control than plaque scores, because many patients brush immediately prior to dental appointments. Baseline investigations that should be undertaken after a BPE to screen for disease in the young patient are summarised in Fig 8-3.

Box 8-3

Marginal gingival bleeding score

- *Place periodontal probe in gingival sulcus and run gently around gingival margin*

- *Four sites for each tooth (buccal, mesial, distal, palatal)*

- *Record presence of bleeding from marginal gingival tissues*

- *Calculate number of bleeding sites as a percentage of overall sites (four for each tooth)*

Plaque score

- *Disclose plaque*

- *Four sites for each tooth (buccal, mesial, distal, palatal)*

- *Record presence of plaque at gingival margin (Fig 8-4)*

- *Calculate number of sites with plaque as a percentage of overall sites (Four for each tooth)*

By subtracting the percentage of sites with marginal gingival bleeding or plaque from 100% these indices can be converted into marginal gingival bleeding-free scores and plaque-free scores (see section on Motivation).

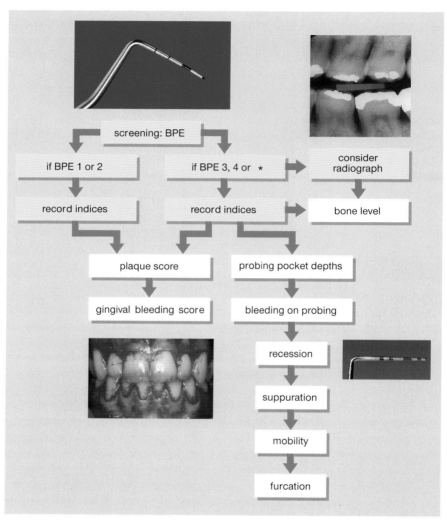

Fig 8-3 Periodontal indices after Basic Periodontal Examination (BPE) screening.

Patient Plaque Control

Parental assistance

A child under the age of seven does not have the manual dexterity to brush their teeth effectively. Therefore, the parent should be shown how to brush the child's teeth. As young children can be fiercely independent, it may be

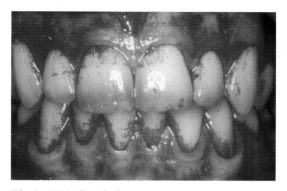

Fig 8-4 Disclosed plaque.

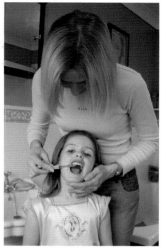

Fig 8-5 Adult brushing a child's teeth.

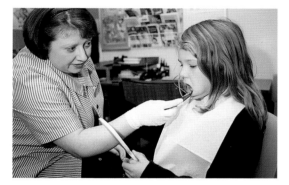

Fig: 8-6 Oral health educator demonstrating brushing.

that the child is encouraged to start the brushing process and then explain to them that the parent will help "get to the fiddly bits". The parent should stand behind with the child standing against the parent's legs (Fig 8-5). The parent can then brush the teeth from behind the child by leaning forwards slightly. Older children can brush their own teeth, however, parental supervision can help to make sure the teeth are brushed for sufficient time and thoroughly.

Disclosing agents
Disclosing agents can increase the effectiveness of tooth brushing, in particular, if their use has been demonstrated in the dental surgery (Fig 8-6). Recording a plaque score as part of the baseline measures can illustrate to the child and parent where the plaque is and the degree of brushing required to remove it.

143

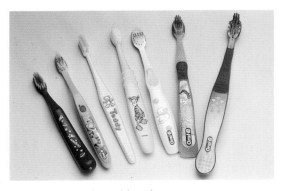

Fig 8-7 Manual toothbrushes.

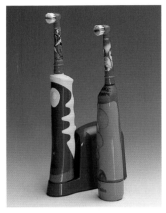

Fig 8-8 Powered tooth-brushes.

Toothbrushes and brushing techniques

A wide range of toothbrushes is available catering for different ages. The tooth-brushes aimed at children and adolescents are usually colourful and may sport popular cartoon characters to make them appealing to the user (Fig 8-7). The scrub tooth brushing technique is effective in children and adolescents; the modified Bass technique can be taught to older children and young adults. Powered toothbrushes are very popular with younger patients. A number of models are specifically targeted at children (Fig 8-8). Those with a rotary head movement are more effective than those with a side-to-side motion. There is evidence that powered toothbrushes may be less abrasive than manual brushes and can be useful for children wearing fixed orthodontic appliances.

Interdental cleaning

Periodontal lesions are predominantly interdental. Therefore, interdental cleaning beneath the contact point is important. Use of interdental aids such as floss should be reserved for the adolescent and young adults who will have sufficient manual dexterity to cope with these. One of the advantages of an electric toothbrush is that interdental plaque removal is improved over manual tooth brushing.

Interdental brushes are very useful where embrasures are larger or there are gaps between the teeth. They are popular with patients. The correct size must be identified for each site. The brush should be precurved and inserted so that the curve faces apically to facilitate subgingival cleaning (Fig 8-9).

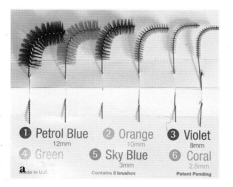
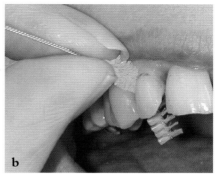

Fig 8-9 (a) Precurved interdental brushes (b) inserted correctly.

Chemical antiplaque agents
Mouth rinses are not indicated in very young children as they are unable to spit out effectively. There is little justification in the literature for the use of antiplaque mouth rinses in adolescents. However, a mouth rinse with fluoride may be indicated for caries prevention in some young patients.

Counselling on Smoking Cessation
Smoking cessation programmes tailored for young people are a high priority due to the growing number of young smokers:
• One in three 15-year old girls in the UK smoke (based on 1996 data).
• On average 11% of boys and 15% of girls aged 11–15 smoke.

Specific leaflets and web resources are available for young smokers (Fig 8-10). Admission of smoking, evidence of staining or the characteristic odour from a recent cigarette should prompt the clinician to approach the problem sensitively and diplomatically. Brief counselling (less than three minutes) delivered by a health professional may influence up to 2% of patients to stop smoking. This figure may seem low, but on a national basis it represents a substantial number. Quit rates can be improved by a follow-up with more intensive advice and support provided by other healthcare workers.

Professional Cleaning
Scaling and prophylaxis are required to remove supragingival stains, plaque and calculus, and subgingival deposits. The term root surface debridement

145

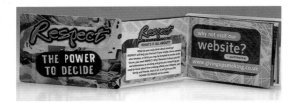

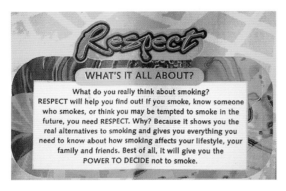

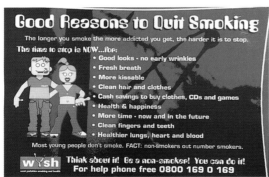

Fig 8-10 (a–c) Smoking cessation leaflets.

(RSD) refers to the removal of subgingival plaque, calculus and endotoxin-associated cementum to leave a biologically inert root surface onto which healing can occur. Subgingival scaling is used to describe removal of subgingival plaque and calculus. Since it is not possible clinically to detect whether or not endotoxin-associated cementum has been detoxified, the distinction between the two terms is often a difficult concept to understand. RSD effectively involves a light but systematic instrumentation of the entire affected root surface, which is far more time consuming than subgingival scaling. RSD has replaced the term root planing, which is a more aggressive, (nonetheless effective) procedure, but conserves less cementum than RSD. The term root surface instrumentation (RSI) will be used in this text to encompass both procedures, but current thinking is that the RSD-approach is the more conservative of viable cementum.

How much scaling can be done in an appointment?
This is a difficult question to answer as it is dependent on many factors. Young patients with little dental experience will benefit from initial visits being kept short, with limited achievable treatment aims to build confidence. A single visit of cleaning may be sufficient for a patient with chronic gingivitis and light supragingival deposits. However, greater time must be allowed for RSI of multiple deep sites.

Use of Local Analgesia
Local analgesia should be used as appropriate when debriding deep sites. This makes the procedure more tolerable for the patient and vasoconstrictor can help to reduce bleeding and the operative field is clearer. Local analgesia is discussed in detail in *Practical Dental Local Analgesia* (Meechan 2002).

Topical anaesthetic agents reduce the discomfort of infiltration anaesthesia, but do not decrease the discomfort of deep regional anaesthetic techniques, such as inferior dental nerve blocks. The agent may need to be left in place for at least five minutes to achieve effect.

Buccal infiltrations are used to achieve analgesia of the upper teeth. In young children and possibly adolescents and young adults the mandibular bone is less dense and lower buccal infiltrations can produce effective soft tissue and pulpal analgesia. Buccal infiltrations may be considered as an alternative to an inferior dental nerve block for lower posterior teeth where isolated pockets are present, and only soft tissue analgesia is required.

Intrapapillary injections produce palatal analgesia. They also help to control local haemorrhage. The needle is inserted at the buccal aspect of the papilla about 2mm apical to the tip of the papilla. Only a small amount of solution (about 0.1ml) is required and it is injected slowly until the papilla blanches.

Regional nerve block injections such as the inferior dental block can be used to reduce the number of injections required if large areas are to be instrumented.

The "tell-show-do" formula (Chapter 9) is useful in taking a young patient through the experience of an injection. The practitioner shows the patient the cotton wool roll and topical gel and explains the fuzzy feeling it will give. The operator and assistant should control the child's field of vision and distract the child with conversation. The injection may be described as "a spray that is going to spread over the tooth and make the cheek fuzzy". In general, avoid showing the child the needle so as not to provoke anxiety but the initial explanation is important so that the procedure is anticipated and does not come as a surprise or shock.

Instrumentation
The instrumentation techniques and armamentarium for performing periodontal therapy are discussed by Heasman, *et al.* (*Successful Periodontal Therapy: A Non-surgical Approach*, 2004). Powered scalers (ultrasonic and sonic) and area-specific curettes (e.g. Gracey area-specific curettes) are the recommended instruments for younger patients, as they are for adults. It may be necessary, however, to utilise slimline tips for powered scalers and "mini-five" Gracey curettes, which are finer hand instruments, for children and younger adults, to avoid stretching and traumatising the soft tissues.

Extractions
Arrangements should be made to extract teeth with a hopeless prognosis and provide immediate dentures, as required.

Response to Initial Therapy
The response to the initial periodontal therapy is crucial in determining the next phase of treatment. The indices that were recorded at baseline should be repeated 8–12 weeks after completion of initial therapy. Probing should be avoided in the early period following RSI (first six weeks) to avoid disruption of the developing long junctional epithelium and measurement errors related to soft tissue remodelling during healing. Questions that should be posed at this stage are:
- Are the oral hygiene and gingival health satisfactory?
- Has the young patient achieved his or her maximum potential for plaque removal and marginal bleeding-free surfaces?
- Are probing pocket depths 3mm or less and free from bleeding on probing?

If the answers are yes, supportive therapy is required. If no, corrective therapy is required.

Corrective Therapy

The corrective phase of therapy is intended to restore function and aesthetics. At its most simple it entails further non-surgical therapy of non-responsive sites. It may, however, involve the use of surgical therapy or of antimicrobial adjuncts. The main areas of corrective therapy are summarised in Fig 8-1.

The Non-Responding Site, Tooth, Mouth and Patient

Non-response can be related to the risk factors for disease in the individual patient presenting at the site, tooth, mouth or patient level (see Chapple and Gilbert 2002). Although only 20–30% of sites that bleed on probing will go on to show further deterioration, bleeding on probing from the base of the pocket is suggestive of a non-responding site, particularly if combined with a pocket of the same depth or greater than was charted at baseline. In a patient who smokes, bleeding on probing can be masked, placing greater emphasis on probing pocket depth measures to evaluate individual sites. In contrast, in a non-smoker, a pocket that remains the same depth after treatment, but no longer bleeds on probing can be considered to have responded to therapy. A site showing suppuration can be considered as non-responding.

Teeth that have developed furcation involvement or increased mobility may be non-responsive. However, other factors must be evaluated carefully. Recession as part of healing may have exposed a furcation defect and mobility may have increased if large supragingival calculus deposits were initially "splinting" a tooth. The eventual mobility of a tooth will be related to the amount of residual periodontal support and occlusal forces, but mobility may remain in the presence of a healthy but reduced periodontium.

A mouth may not respond well to treatment if oral hygiene has been poor. A patient may not respond if they are a smoker or have a systemic disease such as diabetes that is poorly controlled.

Non-surgical or Surgical Therapy?

Non-surgical therapy is generally very effective for periodontal diseases. It is relatively atraumatic and can be repeated as required. It is tolerated well by patients and can be provided by hygienists as well as by dentists. Although there may be some recession following treatment, this is less than following surgical techniques. The effectiveness of treatment is largely dependent on the rigour of the patient's daily plaque control regime. However, non-surgical therapy may not achieve thorough root debridement when:

- there is reduced access to a pocket
- pockets are deep (greater than 6mm)
- furcation involvement is present or
- anatomical features limit access.

Other factors such as the time spent on a site and the experience of the operator will also influence the effectiveness of non-surgical instrumentation. In view of the above, further non-surgical therapy is usually the first line in management of any non-responding sites, in particular, if any residual subgingival calculus deposits can be detected.

A surgical approach to debridement should be considered if it will provide improved access for calculus removal. Periodontal surgery to access deep pockets can be useful in the management of aggressive periodontitis. It may be undertaken with or without adjunctive antimicrobial therapy (see later). On its own it has been shown to be successful in reducing *A. actinomycetemcomitans*, a key pathogen in the localised form of aggressive periodontitis. Periodontal surgery can also be undertaken to:

- regenerate periodontal tissues
- restore function and aesthetics in patients with gingival overgrowth
- provide a tissue contour that facilitates a patient's plaque control
- correct mucogingival deformities (recession defects) or to prevent such defects where it is anticipated that they may develop (e.g. prior to specific orthodontic tooth movements).

Recession can generally be managed by non-surgical periodontal therapy and prevention of further progression by identifying and eliminating, where possible, any aetiological factors (see review by Tugnait and Clerehugh, 2001). Surgical techniques may be used where the condition is progressive or where modification of an aetiological factor (such as a high fraenum that is impeding oral hygiene) can be anticipated to stabilise the condition. Patients for whom some type of periodontal surgery may be an appropriate option should be referred to a specialist periodontist for treatment.

Systemic Antimicrobial Therapy
Systemic antimicrobial therapy is not indicated in patients with chronic periodontitis, even if this presents in the adolescent or young adult. It may be indicated in patients with aggressive periodontitis. Often the practitioner will have referred such a patient for specialist care, but it may be appropriate for a course of initial therapy to have been provided in the general practice setting. The response to initial therapy in a patient with aggressive dis-

ease will often be monitored earlier than for most patients (six to eight weeks after completion of therapy). Non-responding sites should be re-instrumented and adjunctive systemic antimicrobials considered when the overall mass of microbial plaque and calculus has been reduced. Systemic antimicrobial therapy should not be administered without prior or adjunctive mechanical treatment to disrupt the plaque biofilm, since the structure of the biofilm prevents the medication from reaching the target organisms at an effective antimicrobial dose. There is no consensus regarding the optimum choice of drug. Four regimes that have been shown to have clinical benefit in localised aggressive disease are:

- Tetracycline (250mg) four times daily for 21 days; the alternative use of doxycycline (200mg loading dose then 100mg daily for 20 days) is a more convenient regimen, but there is less consistent evidence of efficacy.
- Metronidazole (200mg) three times daily for 10 days.
- Metronidazole (200mg) and amoxycillin (250mg) three times daily for seven days. This is a most effective regimen due to the synergistic effect of the two antibiotics and their hydroxymetabolites.
- Augmentin (Co-amoxiclav) 375mg three times daily for 10 days (private prescription needed).

These regimes and doses are suitable for patients over 12 years of age. Doses for younger children can be found in the current *Dental Practitioners' Formulary* provided by the British Dental Association and Royal Pharmaceutical Society of Great Britain. It is important to note that the best results are reported when the mechanical therapy is started and completed during the dosing period.

Local Antimicrobial Therapy

A number of local antimicrobial agents are available for the treatment of chronic periodontitis in adults. Clinically, local antimicrobials have shown a small benefit in comparison to non-surgical therapy alone. Local antimicrobials may have a role in the management of persistent deep pockets in smokers for whom surgery is not recommended because of their habit. However, the use of local antimicrobials in the management of chronic periodontitis in young patients has not specifically been explored and there is little evidence to support their use in this age group.

Additional Treatments

The corrective phase of therapy seeks to provide definitive treatment to optimise the function and aesthetics of the dentition. Consideration may be

151

given at this stage to orthodontic therapy and advanced restorative treatment where appropriate. When bone loss is severe teeth may drift leading to "flaring", diastema, rotation, extrusion, tipping and midline shift. Orthodontic realignment can be considered, provided the periodontal condition has been brought under control. Care must be taken when orthodontically moving teeth that have reduced bone support and a thorough supportive programme should be in place while treatment is being carried out.

Replacement of lost teeth may be required at this stage with immediate dentures being exchanged for definitive dentures or bridges. The quality and quantity of the residual periodontal support of potential abutment and load bearing teeth needs careful evaluation. In general the placement of restorations with minimal encroachment on gingival margins will give the best outcome for long-term periodontal health. This is of particular importance in the young patient.

Supportive Therapy and Recall

The aims of supportive therapy, formerly called "maintenance therapy", are to:
• Prevent the recurrence and progression of disease in patients who have been treated previously for periodontal disease.
• Prevent or reduce the incidence of tooth loss.
• Increase the probability of locating and treating other diseases that are found within the oral cavity.

The key factors in supportive therapy are summarised in Fig 8-1.

Compliance
Good patient compliance is fundamental to a favourable outcome of periodontal treatment. It is therefore important to assess how well the patient is co-operating with homecare regimes and smoking cessation advice where indicated. Compliance in attending for treatment and recall schedules is also essential. Discussion with the patient and parent or guardian may help to identify the cause of any non-attendances for which external factors may be to blame. A supportive but realistic appraisal of attendance is required. The patient and parent or guardian need to be clearly aware of their role and the limitations placed on successful treatment by less than wholehearted involvement.

Plaque Control

If plaque levels are not well controlled periodontal diseases recur. Unfortunately, good plaque control is difficult to achieve. Even the most enthusiastic patient is likely to become less fastidious at cleaning their teeth as time goes on unless they can be remotivated on a regular basis. Therefore, one of the cornerstones of supportive therapy is to encourage the patient to keep their mouth clean and to arrange regular (three to four monthly) recalls.

For the young patient long-term health benefits are difficult to identify with, and therefore less useful as motivating factors to influence behaviour. Brushing charts can be a useful motivating tool for children. These can be prominently displayed at home and serve to remind the child and parent about brushing. Stars can be stuck onto the chart for each brushing episode and this sort of system has been found to be good at engaging the interest of both the child and the parent. An additional option is for the child to receive from the parent a small reward for a week's successful brushing as a further incentive. This has also been used in school-based projects when, of course, there are the added advantages of participation by the child's teachers with further reinforcement of the oral hygiene message at school and shared involvement of the child's peer group.

Periodic use of disclosing tablets can also help support home cleaning and improve its effectiveness. Visits to the dental practice are used to motivate the patient to keep their mouth plaque-free. It is obviously important that whilst oral hygiene advice is reinforced it does not:
• become repetitive
• become boring
• be perceived by the young patient as a telling off.

It is a good idea to encourage the patient to bring his/her own toothbrush when reviewing the effectiveness of tooth brushing. The success of previous advice should be reviewed and changes may be necessary; for instance, the switch from a manual toothbrush to an electric toothbrush may increase motivation and the effectiveness of plaque removal. Disclosing agents and repeated recording of a plaque score will enable an objective assessment of oral hygiene to be made.

Smoking Cessation

A follow-up of any smoking cessation advice should be made at this stage. The young patient should be encouraged in any efforts made to seek the assistance of other health workers and to reduce or quit their habit.

Assessment of Treatment

The indices recorded as part of the initial therapy should now be repeated to determine the outcome of the previous treatment phases. The decision to re-treat a site is based on these clinical findings. Options for treatment include further non-surgical or surgical therapy and follow the principles described earlier in this chapter under "Initial therapy" and "Corrective therapy". It is essential that the **dentist** carry out the assessment of treatment outcomes so that treatment planning can be carried out. Risk analysis at the tooth and specific site levels are necessary at this stage to determine potential reasons for non-responder sites. If further oral hygiene advice or treatment is required, then this can be undertaken by the oral health educator, hygienist or dentist as necessary.

Recall

Recall visits every four to six months may be suitable for most young patients who have been successfully treated for gingivitis or incipient chronic periodontitis. Frequency of recall should be determined on an individual basis, take into account the diagnosis, risk factors and patient motivation and compliance. Many studies have supported the efficacy of supportive therapy in reducing the progression of gingivitis to periodontitis, and reducing attachment and tooth loss. Longitudinal monitoring of the patient's periodontal condition is achieved by repeating the indices (see Initial therapy) at recall visits. This helps to identify persistent problem areas and the overall response to therapy.

Patients with a history of progressing periodontal disease or systemic risk factors may need a shorter recall interval (two to three months). The aggressive forms of periodontitis need more vigilance and, since the return to pre-treatment pathogen levels may take only 9–11 weeks, recall intervals should not normally exceed three months until there is evidence of sustained stability. Supportive therapy can generally be appropriately delivered to such patients in the general dental practice setting, once the corrective phase of therapy has been completed by a specialist. Although the specialist may wish to see the patient in the early part of the supportive phase, to confirm stability of the disease process, the general practitioner is best placed to provide long-term follow-up within the context of caring for the patient's complete oral health.

Management of Acute Periodontal Conditions

Acute episodes lead to an interruption of the planned treatment. This section outlines the management of the following specific conditions (as described in Chapter 5):

- Necrotising periodontal diseases (necrotising ulcerative gingivitis (NUG) and necrotising ulcerative periodontitis (NUP)).
- Periodontal abscess.
- Periodontitis associated with endodontic lesions.

Necrotising Ulcerative Gingivitis

NUG should be treated by local measures to remove gross deposits. The ultrasonic scaler is useful for this purpose. An oxidising mouth rinse (hydrogen peroxide) or chlorhexidine mouth rinse can be prescribed to reduce plaque levels. The patient should be encouraged to use oral hygiene measures, albeit gently in view of the soreness of the gingivae. A systemic antimicrobial agent such as metronidazole (200mg three times daily for three days) is effective at targeting the anaerobic pathogens. When the pain has subsided, thorough initial phase periodontal therapy should be instituted including smoking cessation advice and review of other predisposing factors such as stress. Post healing, significant gingival deformities can be surgically modified as part of the corrective phase of treatment, if they are impeding oral hygiene measures.

Necrotising Ulcerative Periodontitis

NUP is a rare condition associated with HIV infection or other immunocompromised states. Conventional initial therapy should be employed to remove plaque and calculus but it may become necessary to remove necrotic soft tissue and bone. Daily chlorhexidine mouth rinses will help control plaque and metronidazole will also be required to control the infection. Referral of such cases is appropriate.

Periodontal Abscess

A periodontal abscess may present without drainage of pus or with pus draining. If it is not possible to achieve drainage then management includes:

- Relief of occlusion (by grinding the affected or opposing tooth), systemic antimicrobials (metronidazole or penicillin) and painkillers as appropriate.

If pus is ready to drain then management in the acute phase involves:
- achieving drainage:

- local debridement
- incision and drainage.
- hot salt mouth rinses:
  - half teaspoon of salt in cup of hot water
  - rinse for one minute until tumbler emptied, repeat two to three hourly.
- relieve occlusion
- painkillers as appropriate
- review after a few days.

Further periodontal management will be required subsequently at which time the prognosis of the tooth should be evaluated. If there is evidence of systemic involvement then adjunctive systemic antibiotics are indicated for the minimum time until symptoms resolve. Metronidazole (200mg three times daily for three days), penicillin (250mg four times daily for up to 5–7 days), or a combination of metronidazole (200mg) and amoxycillin (250mg) three times daily can be prescribed.

Periodontitis Associated with Endodontic Lesions

This may present with acute symptoms, but can be quiescent. The lesions have a combined aetiology and are commonly referred to as periodontal-endodontic (perio-endo) lesions. Endodontics should be undertaken first and then followed by thorough periodontal therapy. Critical evaluation of the prognosis of the involved tooth should be made before embarking on treatment. Where there is extensive loss of bone support, the prognosis is often poor and extraction is the most appropriate method of management (this is discussed in more detail by Heasman, *et al.*, 2004).

Key Points

- Periodontal therapy can be organised in three phases:
  - initial
  - corrective
  - supportive.
- Baseline measurements give a record of extent of disease and patient plaque control.
- Subsequent measurements:
  - enable response to treatment to be assessed
  - allow detailed planning for advanced treatment
  - help to plan long term maintenance of the periodontal tissues.
- Acute periodontal lesions are managed by relief of pain followed by treatment according to the specific presenting condition.

References

Tugnait A, Clerehugh V. Gingival recession – its significance and management. J Dent 2001;29:381–394.

Further Reading

Chapple ILC, Gilbert AD. Understanding Periodontal Diseases: Assessment and Diagnostic Procedures in Practice. London: Quintessence, 2002.

Heasman PA, Preshaw PM, Robertson P. Successful Periodontal Therapy: A Non-Surgical Approach. London: Quintessence, 2003.

Meechan JG. Practical Dental Local Anaesthesia. London: Quintessence, 2002.

Noble S, Kellett M, Chapple ILC. Decision-Making for the Periodontal Team. London: Quintessence, 2003.

Chapter 9
Communication

Aims

This chapter outlines the key factors that underpin successful communication between patients, parents and members of the dental team, when managing periodontal diseases in children, adolescents and young adults.

Outcome

Having read this chapter the practitioner should have an insight into the development of a child's skills of reasoning and how this impacts upon communication with the child in a dental setting. The role of the parent or guardian in shaping behaviour and supporting dental health objectives should also be appreciated. The practitioner should be aware of effective methods of verbal and written communication for different age groups and of key messages appropriate for children and adolescents, their parents, and young adults.

Introduction

"You must be able to communicate with people in order to be a good dentist." This is a statement to which most of us would subscribe; yet there is a tendency to think that the ability to communicate well is a personality trait. Certainly, some people find it easier than others but, nonetheless, communicating skills can be learnt and developed.

In the context of this book, three-way communication between the dentist, patient and parent is essential and is, of course, fundamental to the workings of the whole dental team. When dealing with children, adolescents and young adults effective communication and treatment planning must take into account the patient's level of development (both mental and physical) and past dental experience. It is not the intention of this chapter to explore stages of development or behavioural management in detail. This is covered in *Child Taming: How to Cope with Children in Dental Practice* (Chadwick and Hosey, 2003).

159

Communication with the Young Patient

The Developing Child

When dealing with the child patient it is important to be aware of the child's capabilities and understanding in order to tailor treatment appropriately.

- Children under seven years tend to be egocentric in their thinking and unable to grasp another person's viewpoint.
- Children under seven years of age may miss many sites in the mouth if brushing unaided and will swallow much of the toothpaste.
- By age seven, children have the motor skills to brush their teeth reasonably well though parental assistance is still valuable.
- Children aged seven – 11 can apply reasoning and consider another person's point of view.
- Children aged 11 upwards will be able to think in a more abstract way, consider different possibilities for action and weigh up alternatives.
- Adolescents tend to be influenced by their peer group.
- Adolescents are not driven by remote goals such as future disease prevention.

Communicating with the Child Patient

When interacting with the child patient it is important that most of the communication is directly with the child – not over their head with the accompanying adult. Care must be taken with choice of language. Jargon should be avoided. As young children do not appreciate the world from anyone else's viewpoint these explanations should be centred on the child and should be accessible, but without being patronising. It is also important that the practitioner addresses the child directly and makes eye contact, even if further explanations then need to be made to the accompanying adult. The dentist may seem more approachable to the child if he or she makes him/herself accessible by sitting, kneeling or squatting down to meet the child at eye level.

It is important to know how a child likes to be addressed and to record that information for future visits. At the beginning of the visit the initial chat should include non-dental topics and this is the time when the patient's level of anxiety about the visit can be gauged. A simple explanation of the intentions of that visit should be given with limited detail, since the exact nature of the appointment may not be determined until the examination. It is important to continue to keep in verbal contact with the patient during the examination. A clear end should be made to the visit and a small reward, such as a sticker, can be given to a young child (Fig 9-1).

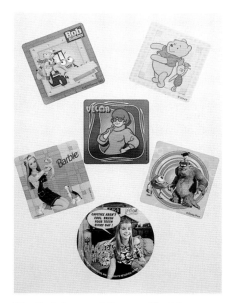

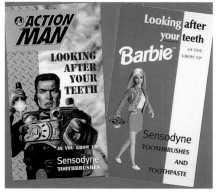

Fig 9-1 Assorted "reward" stickers.

Fig 9-2 Action Man™ and Barbie™ leaflets for children.

When communicating with a child or adolescent patient it is important to tailor your explanations to the individual. Verbal advice can be supplemented by written advice. Commercially produced leaflets and stickers are available that are specifically targeted at different age groups. These are designed to be visually appealing and often use characters with which the child is familiar (Fig 9-2). Children develop at different rates and may appear more or less mature than their years. As children of seven – 11 years of age can apply reasoning, the clinician may be able to link concepts such as plaque with disease, or brushing with health in this age group. Children older than 11 years of age can compare different options and, therefore, can be significantly involved in planning treatment. Oral hygiene techniques are covered in Chapter 8. However, simple take-home messages on gingivitis and chronic periodontitis for children are shown in Box 9-1. Caries prevention advice should also be given in simple terms.

Box 9-1

Information for a Child

Gingivitis

- *Food and bugs (a mixture called plaque) are sticking to your teeth*
- *Plaque can damage your teeth and is making your gums bleed*
- *Plaque is dirty and can make your mouth smell funny*
- *Brushing your teeth makes your mouth feel clean*
- *Brushing makes your teeth and gums strong*
- *Mum/dad (other) may have to brush the tricky bits in your mouth*
- *The dentist, mum and dad, teachers, etc. will be pleased with you for brushing your teeth*
- *We can tell your gums are well (healthy, strong) when they don't bleed when you brush your teeth*

Chronic Periodontitis

- *Food and bugs (a mixture called plaque) are sticking to your teeth*
- *Plaque and hard plaque (tartar/calculus) is making your gums bleed*
- *Plaque and hard plaque (tartar/calculus) is slowly damaging the part of the gum that holds your teeth in your mouth*
- *We can mend your gums by getting your mouth clean*
- *You need to clean the soft plaque away every morning and evening*
- *The dentist (hygienist) will clean the hard plaque away*

Communicating with Adolescent Patients

Adolescent patients are a difficult group to influence on health matters that will affect them in later life. Since they are not driven by remote goals they do not tend to consider how their current behaviour might pose a threat in the longer term. Explanations of health and disease and its consequences should reflect the motivation of teenagers. As peer group acceptance and appearance are far stronger motivation factors, these can be used to engage the interest of the adolescent patient and make the health message pertinent

TOOTH CARE
Update

How kissable are you?
A teenagers' guide to good mouthcare

No 13

Looking after your teeth contributes to the way you look. Sparkling clean, even teeth look good, so you can smile with confidence. Good mouthcare keeps your breath fresh too!

■ **Its over to you**
Nobody wants to lose a tooth from decay or have bleeding gums. Good habits keep tooth decay and gum disease at bay. This way you will ensure that you look and feel good now, and you will keep your teeth for life.

■ **The root of the problem**
Plaque is a sticky substance that develops on the teeth continuously and contains a host of bacteria. These bacteria are the common link between tooth decay, gum disease and bad breath.
The plaque bacteria use the sugars from our food and drink to cause acid attack on the teeth. If this occurs often, then over time, tooth decay or cavities will form. Gum disease is caused when the bacteria infect the gums, causing them to bleed. In the early stages, it is easy to get rid of (by

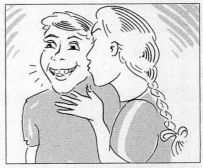

thorough toothbrushing), but if allowed to develop, deep pockets can occur between the tooth and the gum, making the tooth loose and likely to fall out. The smell of gas produced by the activity of the bacteria living in the mouth is the main cause of bad breath! The regular removal of plaque helps fight against all of these problems

■ **To keep plaque at bay you need**

● **Fluoride toothpaste** - fluoride helps to strengthen the tooth against acid attacks. Check that your toothpaste contains fluoride. Toothpastes that

Fig 9-3 Front cover of "Kissable" leaflet for adolescents.

163

to them as individuals. Getting across the message that dental disease may cause bad breath or make a person unattractive is likely to be a more powerful influencing factor than the consequences of periodontal disease or caries. A leaflet that asks how kissable the adolescent might be and subliminally accesses issues of self-esteem and attraction to the opposite sex is shown in Fig 9-3. Leaflets using a photomontage style and romantic storyline, similar to the layout of many teenage magazines, have also been well received by adolescent school children (Fig 9-4a,b). Examples of an explanation to adolescents of the key points of gingivitis and chronic periodontitis are shown in Box 9-2.

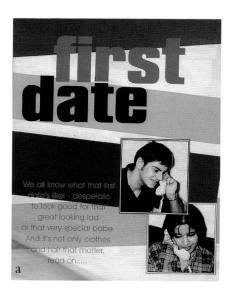

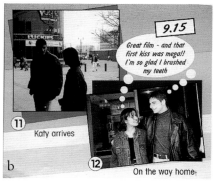

Fig 9-4 (a,b) Photomontage leaflets for adolescents.

Box 9-2

Information for an Adolescent

Gingivitis

- *Food and bugs (a mixture called plaque) are sticking to your teeth*

- *Plaque is making your gums bleed and has given you some gum disease*

- *Plaque and gum disease can make your breath smell and other people will notice this (especially if they get up close!)*

- *You could even lose teeth and have gaps showing if gum disease gets really bad*

- *Brushing your teeth will make your mouth feel clean and your breath fresh*

- *Brushing can make your gums strong and keep your teeth white*

- *Careful brushing will help to stop your gums bleeding and stop that gum disease*

- *Everyone notices an attractive, healthy smile!*

Chronic Periodontitis

- *Food and bugs (a mixture called plaque) are sticking to your teeth*

- *Plaque and hard plaque (tartar/calculus) is making your gums bleed*

- *Plaque and hard plaque (tartar/calculus) has got under the gum and is slowly damaging the parts that hold your teeth in your mouth*

- *If the process carries on eventually your teeth could get loose or could fall out*

- *Your gums can be healed by getting your mouth clean*

- *You will need to clean the soft plaque away every morning and evening*

- *The dentist (hygienist) will clean the hard plaque away*

Tell–Show–Do and Positive Reinforcement

The degree of experience of a child patient is substantially less than that of an adult. Much about dental treatment and the dental surgery environment may be unfamiliar to young patients. The principle behind the "tell-show-do" method is to familiarise the child with a procedure. A task can be broken down into small achievable parts to allow the child to build up confidence in themselves and the clinician. An example of using the tell-show-do technique is shown in Box 9-3. If necessary, the task can be broken down further for a nervous child. Other non-threatening stages can be added which involve the child and build up their confidence, including getting them to hold a large mirror to see or count their teeth or to hold the toothpaste (polish) container. It is useful to get the child involved in small decisions so that they can feel in control. Try to ask them questions that allow you to carry out the intended procedure and do not give the child the option of refusing it. For example, rather than asking the child: "Can I polish your teeth?" the dentist can ask which of two colours or flavours of toothpaste should be used to clean the child's teeth. Bear in mind that two options give a choice, but many options may simply be counterproductive and delay the process.

Box 9-3

Tell–Show–Do

"I am going to clean your teeth with a special electric toothbrush"

> *Show disconnected slow-speed hand piece attachment with rubber cup or brush attached*

"Let me show you how the brush works"

"Let's try the brush on my fingernail"

> *Demonstrate disconnected brush manually on your own fingernail (without gloves)*

"Let's try the brush on your fingernail"

> *Demonstrate disconnected brush manually on child's fingernail*

"It's an electric toothbrush so I'm going to plug it in"

"It makes a great whizzy noise! Shall I go fast or slow with it?"

> *Connect slow-speed hand piece and demonstrate away from patient so child can hear the noise*

"Let's brush it on my fingernail, it tickles a bit!"

> *Demonstrate on your own fingernail*

"Let's try it on your fingernail and see how ticklish you are"

> *Demonstrate on child's fingernail*

"Have you got ticklish teeth? Let's see if you have."

> *Demonstrate on child's tooth*

The child's trust in the dentist will increase if a pact is made to stop the examination or procedure at a prearranged signal such as the lifting of the child's arm. Having made this agreement it is important that the dentist strictly observes it to build the child's confidence. Often the child will test the dentist early in the procedure to check that the arrangement is bona fide. However, once reassured the signal is generally infrequently used. Therefore, when it may not be possible to stop immediately this should be explained to the patient in advance. For example, you may say that the cleaner that you will be using sprays lots of water and you will have to switch it off first before taking it out of the mouth, otherwise the child and dentist will get very wet. However, you will remove the cleaner as soon as possible after the child's signal. This method can be very effective even in quite nervous youngsters.

Positive reinforcement should be used to praise and encourage good aspects of the child's behaviour. In a visit that did not achieve all its goals, it is usually possible to identify some aspect such as a fleeting opening of the mouth that can be welcomed and praised, even if was insufficient for the intended dental task. Details of other methods of dealing with anxious patients, including pharmacological approaches, can be found in a paediatric dentistry textbook (see Further reading).

Communication with Young Adult Patients

The young adult's level of understanding and reasoning enables the dentist to give a more detailed explanation of disease processes and their consequences. Nevertheless, the young adult may not readily accept the personal relevance of current behaviour to disease outcomes when the health detriment lies many years into the future. As a result, the young adult may not fully accept an active role in disease prevention or management. Also peer pressure can still be an influential factor in behaviour, for example, in smoking or attendance for regular dental check-ups. For many people motivation for oral health is related to appearance, attractiveness and self-esteem rather than pure health goals. Examples of the key points in an explanation of aggressive periodontitis to young adults are shown in Box 9-4. Additional smoking cessation advice will be necessary where the habit is a contributory factor.

Box 9-4

Information About Aggressive Periodontitis for a Young Adult

- *Part of the gum attachment and bone that holds your teeth in your mouth has become damaged*

- *A number of different factors, some of which we can't explain, have made you prone to this gum disease*

- *Although plaque and tartar are not the only cause they have contributed to this gum disease*

- *The gum disease is of concern as it has started early in your life and seems to be progressing rapidly*

- *If the gum disease goes untreated you are in danger of developing loose teeth, widening spaces between your teeth or even losing teeth*

- *You can have treatment which will try to slow down or stop the disease*

- *Treatment involves the dentist/hygienist reducing the bugs that live in plaque and tartar below the gum by scaling*

- *AND alongside this you will need to remove the plaque thoroughly above the gum line for the treatment to work*

- *Additional treatment measures may include a course of antibiotics*

Communication with the Parent: The Parent's Role

Parents or guardians can shape their children's attitudes to dentistry; for example, a child who has never personally had a bad dental experience can attend a dental surgery full of anxiety fuelled by the family's perception of dental treatment. If the parent's support is gained then this can have a very positive impact on treatment outcomes. Parents can reinforce the oral hygiene advice that is given as part of the periodontal management, supervise home disclosing of plaque and tooth brushing, and praise the child's efforts. Parental attitudes, e.g. making the time to check their child's brushing can influence how often a child brushes. Parents can also positively reinforce the oral health message given in the practice by using brushing charts with stars or other rewards to maintain a child's interest and encourage compliance.

Many leaflets are available for parents to gain information about their children's oral health. Leaflets that are perceived as relevant have more chance of success, so it is worthwhile displaying a variety of these in the practice for babies, toddlers as well as for older children (Fig 9-5). Take-home messages for parents on gingivitis and chronic periodontitis in their child are shown in Box 9-5.

Box 9-5

Information For the Parent

Gingivitis

- *Gum disease occurs in children*

- *Plaque (a mixture of food and bugs) causes gum disease as well as decay*

- *Limited damage to your child's gums has occurred so far*

- *Careful brushing can get rid of the plaque and the gum disease*

- *Children need an adult's help with brushing to reach awkward areas*

- *Try to supervise your child's brushing*

Chronic Periodontitis

- *Plaque and tartar have damaged part of the gum attachment and bone that holds the teeth in the mouth*

- *If damage continues teeth can eventually become loose and be lost*

- *The disease has been picked up early so little damage has occurred so far*

- *The damage is of concern in a young person whose teeth should last for many years to come*

- *The disease can be stopped by cleaning treatment to remove the tartar and by plaque removal at home*

- *You can help your child by supervising brushing (so plaque is removed thoroughly) and by bringing them for treatment*

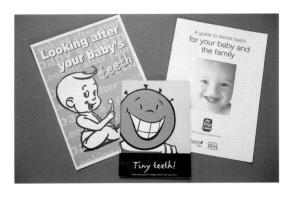

Fig 9-5 Leaflets for parents.

The dentist has to be sensitive to other relevant issues, with which the parent may be faced. The parent may feel guilty about their child's dental health especially if they believe it was an omission on their part that has contributed to the problem, or they may be angry that the disease was not identified earlier. Some periodontal conditions have a genetic component and a parent may be anxious about other family members.

Communication and the Dental Team

Periodontal therapy is best provided by the whole dental team. For this to work well members of the team have to be clear about their role and responsibilities within the team. Good communication between all team members will ensure optimal provision of care for patients. The dentist, who is the team leader, should carry out examination and treatment planning. A dental hygienist may provide several stages of initial therapy. A practice may have other personnel trained as oral health educators who can also be involved in delivery of care. Any professionals complementary to dentistry (PCDs) should be provided with a written prescription by the lead clinician for the treatment they are to undertake. This clarifies the treatment that was intended, any special factors to be taken into consideration when delivering treatment, the length of appointments and indicates at what stage the dentist wishes to review the patient's progress. A simple prescription pro forma can make the job of writing a prescription quick and straightforward. Frequently used treatments can be itemised and the practitioner can ring "Yes" or "No" alternatives to indicate whether or not the treatment is required for the named patient. All staff should be clear how the referring dentist wants to be informed of any new developments or problems in implementing the treatment plan. In a small practice this may be a simple chat between colleagues but in many busy surgeries it is not always possible to speak to someone on demand. A written record has the advantage that the specific details will be available at a later date.

When several members of the team are involved in the provision of treatment the oral health message will be delivered by different methods and in different forms of words. This can positively reinforce a message that can become strengthened simply by virtue of having reached the patient from a number of sources on a number of separate occasions. However, although it is valuable for the patient to be given information by several personnel it is important that the general message is consistent. Part-time team members and new staff need to be updated of any significant shifts in practice policy, for instance in recommending products so that everyone is "singing from the same hymn sheet". The contribution of all members of the team should be recognised and the non-clinical members should not be overlooked. For instance, the receptionist can have a role in the oral health education of patients depending on the practice set-up, by giving out leaflets, dispensing toothbrushes or further praising the child as they return from the dental surgery with a sticker.

An additional member of the dental team, who may be involved in the care of some patients is the specialist periodontist. Good communication between the dentist and specialist is essential so that it is clear which aspects of treatment are to be undertaken in which setting. This is particularly important as periodontal treatment plans can be of lengthy duration. Equally important is that the patient and parent understand how and where care is to be delivered, as confusion can lead to lapses in attendance and suboptimum patient management.

Key Points

- Communication with the child, adolescent and young adult patient should reflect their age, development, understanding and past dental experiences.
- Communication is helped by use of simple language directed at the patient and can be reinforced by targeted written information.
- Motivation should try to harness issues of relevance to the young patient.
- Explanations of disease and treatment should be made to the parents or guardians of child and adolescent patients and their active support encouraged.

- Dental team members should develop and agree a simple practice policy for communication about patient care, including referral and review procedures.

Further Reading

Chadwick, Hosey. Child Taming: How to Cope with Children in Dental Practice. London: Quintessence, 2003.

Welbury RR (Ed.) Paediatric Dentistry. 2nd edn. Oxford: Oxford University Press, 2001.

Chapter 10
Treat or Refer?

Aim

This chapter considers how to assess when younger patients should be treated within a general dental practice setting and when they should be referred for specialist care.

Outcome

Having read this chapter the practitioner should understand which cases can be managed safely in general practice and which should be referred for specialist care. The reader will also have gained knowledge about the appropriate information to include in a referral letter for younger periodontal patients.

Making the Decision to Treat or Refer

The decision to treat or refer a young patient will be dependent on three issues (Fig 10-1):
* the general dental practitioner's expertise
* patient-centred factors
* complexity of the case.

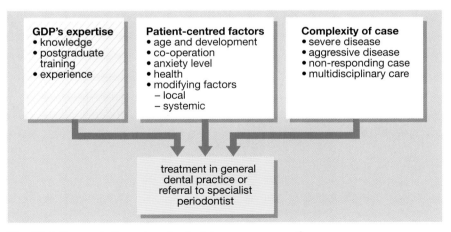

Fig 10-1 Factors influencing the decision to treat or refer.

173

The British Society of Periodontology has developed a referral policy based on a patient having been screened for periodontal diseases using the Basic Periodontal Examination (BPE). Although primarily targeted at adults, the principles described below can be applied successfully to younger patients. Not every patient with the features listed in Box 10-1 will need specialist care; however, the need for referral should be considered for such patients.

Box 10-1

Younger Patients Who May Need Referral

- *Diagnosis of aggressive periodontitis*

- *Incipient chronic periodontitis not responding to non-surgical therapy provided by the practice team*

- *Systemic medical conditions associated with periodontal destruction (see Chapters 5, 7 and 8)*

- *Genetic conditions predisposing to periodontal destruction (Chapter 7)*

- *Drug-induced gingival overgrowth (Chapter 5)*

- *At risk from delivery of periodontal care (e.g. risk of infective endocarditis)*

- *Local factors (e.g. root morphology) affecting prognosis*

- *Requiring evaluation for periodontal surgery*

- *Requiring diagnosis of rare and complex clinical pathology (Chapters 6 and 7)*

- *Requiring complex multidisciplinary medical and dental care*

Another useful service that is provided by specialist periodontists is the provision of a specialist opinion and treatment plan. This may be valuable in the situation in which the dentist is happy to treat the patient but wants confirmation of a diagnosis or assistance with planning the management. The specialist may suggest a division of the therapy between the practice and a specialist centre. This can be particularly helpful when long distances are involved and the patient/parent find it easier to have most of their care delivered locally.

The Referral Process

The Referral Letter

The principal method of referring a patient to a specialist is still via a written referral letter. It has been shown that the quality of referral letters is considerably better when a referral pro forma is used (Snoad et al. 1999). Having a pro forma or some other form of template can prevent key pieces of information from being omitted as well as making the process of writing the letter simpler. An example referral letter is shown in Fig 10-2 highlighting the key points that should be included, although there may be additional details relevant in individual cases which should be added as appropriate. Copies of probing pocket depth and bleeding charts may be of value if these are available.

It is important that the radiation dosage from radiographs is kept as low as possible in children as the tissues of younger people are more radiosensitive than those of adults. To minimise the dose and justify the taking of radiographs it is considered best practice to have available previous radiographs and the practitioner should send relevant radiographs with the referral. Many specialists will specifically ask the referring dentist to forward radiographs if none have been sent with the original letter. Previous radiographs may reduce the need for further films at the consultation visit and may help to assess disease progression if films over a number of years are available. Practitioners may be reluctant to send in radiographs for a number of reasons including their potential loss. It is worthwhile including in the referral letter a specific request for return of the radiographs after their use. Many specialists are able to copy radiographs and return the originals to the practitioner.

Periodontal therapy can be divided into three phases (see Chapter 8): initial, corrective and supportive. It is usually appropriate for management of plaque-induced gingival and periodontal diseases for a course of initial therapy to have been provided and evaluated by the practitioner before taking the decision to refer. However, if the condition is considered aggressive in behaviour the referral may be sent whilst providing the initial therapy. Some of the non-plaque-induced lesions (see Chapters 6 and 7) may, however, require an immediate referral for definitive diagnosis and management in a specialist centre (Fig 10-3).

The Specialist's Reply

In response to the referral letter, the practitioner should receive a reply from the specialist periodontist. This should give a diagnosis and an outline of the treatment plan. While the periodontal therapy is provided in the specialist

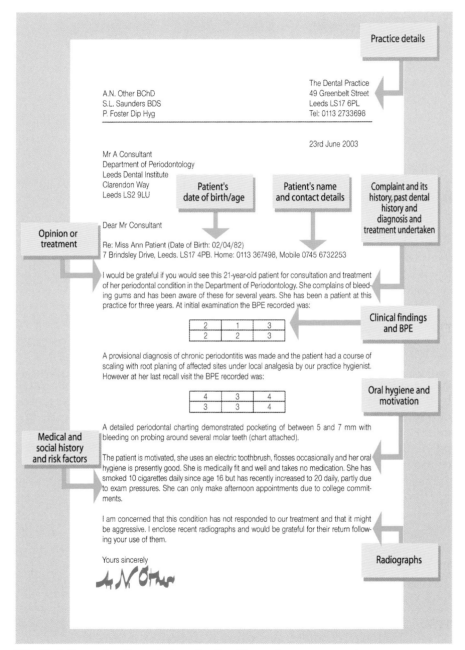

Fig 10-2 Example of a periodontal referral letter for a young patient.

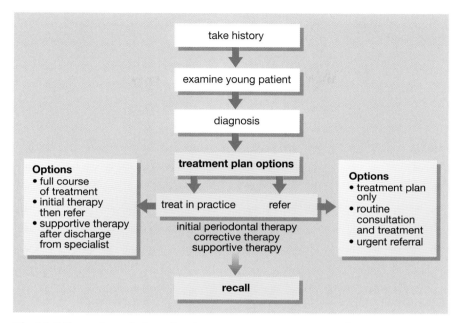

Fig 10-3 Stages in periodontal patient management: treat or refer.

centre the patient's general dental care will normally continue to be provided by the practitioner. In many cases the delivery of the referred patient's periodontal care will be divided between the specialist centre and the general dental practice. The patient will usually receive the initial and supportive phases of therapy in the practice and the corrective therapy in the specialist centre (see Chapter 8).

It is important to remember that waiting lists in hospitals are a reality so treatment may not begin immediately following receipt of the practitioner's letter. The general dental practitioner should therefore continue to provide general periodontal care for the patient until the course of specialist treatment starts. This avoids a hiatus in the patient's periodontal management.

The Dental Team

Who's on the Team?

Although the dental team is a term that has been used for many years it is clear that the composition of the team and individuals, roles within it are changing. The number of practices that employ a dental hygienist continues to increase. Many dental nurses are trained as oral health educators. Specialist practitioners may now be found in the "high street", not just in hospitals. Single-handed practices are less common, with dentists working in group practices often with a practice manager. New dental therapy courses have been established, offering a dual qualification in dental hygiene and therapy and bachelor's degree courses have already been established for some PCDs. All these factors indicate a continued evolution of the dental team and how patient care is best delivered. So who are the members of the dental team (Fig 10-4) as it relates to periodontal care for younger patients in general dental practice? These include the:

- dental nurse
- oral health educator
- dental hygienist
- dental therapist
- dental technician
- clinical dental technician
- receptionist
- practice manager
- general dental practitioner
- specialist periodontist.

The above list is not exhaustive. In addition, the general medical practitioner or other medical specialists may have a role to play in the management of some patients, as may other dental specialists.

Delivery of Care

The general dental practitioner is the dental team leader, responsible for the overall management of the patient's dental care. If a young patient is referred to a specialist then the role of co-ordinating the periodontal therapy will fall to the specialist periodontist. However, the general care of the patient will be provided by the general dental practitioner and close liaison will be needed between the two team members.

Periodontal care is most efficiently delivered by utilising all the appropriate members of the team. The duties of several members of the dental team are expanding (discussed in detail by Noble, et al., 2003). The support members' input includes providing a welcoming and efficient practice environment. The young patient/parent may perceive this in many ways.

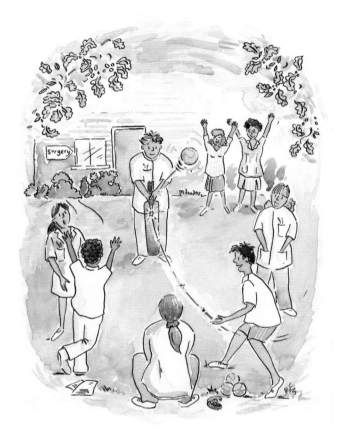

Fig 10-4 The dental team: dental nurse, oral health educator, hygienist, technician, receptionist, practice manager, general dental practitioner, periodontist.

The **receptionist** who was on the other end of a phone when the appointment was made can, on arrival, help to instil confidence and alleviate anxiety. Parents will welcome a tidy and clean waiting area that is child friendly with books or toys that will occupy the child's attention until the appointment is due. Good practice management means the patient notes and radiographs will be at hand and stocks of recommended oral hygiene products are kept up to date.

179

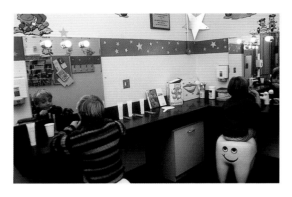

Fig 10-5 Oral hygiene room.

The **dental nurse** can have a range of skills beyond assisting the dentist and can help to manage a child's behaviour. With training in oral health education the dental nurse can be active in promoting dental health and demonstrating brushing and interdental cleaning. This can work to great effect if instruction is given in a dedicated "prevention room" furnished with sink and mirrors, where the child's teeth can be disclosed and help given to clean them (Fig 10-5). Such a non-threatening environment can be valuable in introducing an anxious patient to dentistry, whether a child, adolescent or young adult.

The **dental hygienist** has multiple skills which are useful in the care of periodontal patients. Although the dental team leader must have overall responsibility for the progress of the case, the hygienist will be able to collect information of importance in formulating treatment plans and monitoring progress by recording indices. The hygienist will also be able to carry out non-surgical therapy and use local analgesia where the dentist has prescribed this. The importance of communication between these key team members has been discussed in Chapter 9. Following any treatment by the hygienist arrangements must be in place for the dentist to be able to evaluate the response to treatment. It is not legally acceptable for a patient to have seen the hygienist for scaling before they have been seen for an examination by the dentist.

The **dental technician** may be involved in the periodontal management of a patient if study casts, cast restorations or dentures are required. Designs of restorations and appliances must be sympathetic to the periodontal tissues. Careful contouring of crowns and bridges is required to avoid creating overhanging restorations and for the restoration to be accessible to cleaning. Dentures should have gingival clearance wherever possible and be adequately supported and retained. It is the dentist's responsibility to provide the technician with a good design and clear prescription.

The **dental practitioner** co-ordinates and takes responsibility for the overall care of the patient and the work of the team. The dentist should draw up a clear treatment plan, indicating the parts of the treatment to be carried out by specific team members. If the sequence of appointments is important that should also be made clear to the team, patient and, where appropriate, the parent, as one cancelled appointment can affect the plan. The dentist will assess the patient's response to therapy and determine further treatment needs including the appropriate regime for supportive therapy. The dentist will also undertake extractions, removal of overhanging ledges and provision of fixed and removable restorative work.

The **specialist periodontist** will undertake periodontal treatment planning and necessary therapy for the referred patient and should make clear whether or not any of the procedures in the three phases of therapy are to be provided in the practice. Generally, the practitioner will carry out any restorations that require modification or replacement (to eliminate plaque retention factors). Extraction of teeth with poor prognosis and their replacement with an immediate denture may be required, as part of the periodontal therapy. Such treatment will usually be carried out in the referring practice. Interim appliances may be called for during the periodontal therapy with definitive restorations on completion of the therapy. The specialist may recommend particular designs of denture or fixed restorations for construction and delivery by the practitioner.

Discharge Process from Specialist and Back to the Practitioner

On completion of the corrective phase of therapy the patient will be evaluated and the supportive phase will be planned (see Heasman, *et al.*, 2004). Although the periodontist may wish to see the patient for review of the condition, in most cases the patient will be discharged for supportive care within the general dental practice. The periodontist's letter of discharge should advise the practitioner on aspects of the supportive therapy including the frequency of visits required and teeth or sites requiring specific attention when monitoring.

The practitioner needs to be vigilant for any recurrence of disease or relapse in the patient's homecare. It is all too easy for the patient and parent to think that the periodontal problem has been solved and their efforts can "ease off".

Practitioners can expect to manage the long-term supportive care of patients with both chronic and aggressive disease within their practice. Chapter 8 describes the planning and implementation of supportive therapy. The frequency of recall visits will usually be greater in a patient who has had aggressive disease. Re-referral should be considered if deterioration of the periodontium occurs subsequently.

Key Points

- The decision to treat or refer a patient for periodontal therapy is based on the general practitioner's expertise, patient-centred factors and complexity of the case.
- Administrative information and clinical details with a BPE and relevant radiographs should be included in a periodontal referral letter.
- Many patients with periodontal diseases will be treated in general dental practice.
- Cases that are referred to a specialist periodontist may have initial and supportive phases of their periodontal care carried out in general dental practice.
- Periodontal therapy is best managed by utilising the skills of the entire dental team.

Reference

Snoad RJ, Eaton KA, Furniss JS, Newman HN. Appraisal of a standardised periodontal referral pro forma. Br Dent J 1999;187:42–46.

Further Reading

Heasman PA, Preshaw PM, Robertson P. Successful Periodontal Therapy: A Non-Surgical Approach. London: Quintessence, 2003.

Noble S, Kellet M, Chapple ILC. Decision-Making for the Periodontal Team. London: Quintessence, 2003.

Index

183

Quintessentials for General Dental Practitioners Series

in 36 volumes

Editor-in-Chief: Professor Nairn H F Wilson

The Quintessentials for General Dental Practitioners Series covers basic principles and key issues in all aspects of modern dental medicine. Each book can be read as a stand-alone volume or in conjunction with other books in the series.

Publication date,
approximately

Oral Surgery and Oral Medicine, Editor: John G Meechan

Practical Dental Local Anaesthesia	available
Practical Oral Medicine	Spring 2004
Practical Conscious Sedation	available
Practical Surgical Dentistry	Spring 2004

Imaging, Editor: Keith Horner

Interpreting Dental Radiographs	available
Panoramic Radiology	Spring 2004
Twenty-first Century Dental Imaging	Autumn 2004

Periodontology, Editor: Iain L C Chapple

Understanding Periodontal Diseases: Assessment and Diagnostic Procedures in Practice	available
Decision-Making for the Periodontal Team	available
Successful Periodontal Therapy – A Non-Surgical Approach	available
Periodontal Management of Children, Adolescents and Young Adults	available
Periodontal Medicine: A Window on the Body	Autumn 2005

Implantology, Editor: Lloyd J Searson

Implantology in General Dental Practice	Spring 2004
Managing Orofacial Pain in Practice	Spring 2004

Endodontics, Editor: John M Whitworth

Rational Root Canal Treatment in Practice	available
Managing Endodontic Failure in Practice	Spring 2004
Managing Dental Trauma in Practice	Spring 2004
Preventing Pulpal Injury in Practice	Autumn 2005

Prosthodontics, Editor: P Finbarr Allen

Teeth for Life for Older Adults	available
Complete Dentures – from Planning to Problem Solving	available
Removable Partial Dentures – A Systematic Approach	Spring 2004
Fixed Prosthodontics for the General Dental Practitioner	Autumn 2005
Occlusion: A Theoretical and Team Approach	Autumn 2004

Operative Dentistry, Editor: Paul A Brunton

Decision-Making in Operative Dentistry	available
Applied Dental Materials in Operative Dentistry	Spring 2005
Aesthetic Dentistry	Spring 2004
Indirect Restorations	Autumn 2004
Psychological and Behavioural Management of Adult Dental Patients	Autumn 2004

Paediatric Dentistry/Orthodontics, Editor: Marie Therese Hosey

Child Taming: How to Cope with Children in Dental Practice	available
Paediatric Cariology	Spring 2004
Treatment Planning for the Developing Dentition	Autumn 2004

General Dentistry and Practice Management, Editor: Raj Rattan

The Business of Dentistry	available
Risk Management	Spring 2004
Practice Management for the Dental Team	Autumn 2004
IT in Dentistry: A Working Manual	Autumn 2005
Quality Assurance	Autumn 2004
Dental Practice Design	Spring 2005

Quintessence Publishing Co. Ltd., London